Exploring Well-being

Can we teach others how to lead a fulfilling life? The notion of personal well-being has recently shot up the political and educational agendas, placing the child's well-being at the heart of the school's work.

With his renowned talent for distilling the most complex of philosophical arguments into accessible laymen's terms, John White addresses the maze of issues surrounding well-being, bringing clarity to this dissension and confusion. This accessible book expertly guides you through the conflicting perspectives on well-being found in the educational world by:

- examining religious and secular views of human fulfilment and of a meaningful life;
- analysing the appeal of celebrity, wealth and consumerism to so many of our children;
- asking what role pleasure, success, autonomy, work, life planning and worthwhile activities play in children's flourishing;
- showing how proposals to encourage children's well-being impact on schools' aims and learning arrangements.

Whether you have little background in education and philosophy or are reading as a teacher, student or policy-maker, this engaging book will take you right to the heart of these critical issues. It will leave you with a sharply focused picture of a remodelled educational system fit for the new millennium, committed to helping every child to enjoy a fulfilling life.

John White is Emeritus Professor of Philosophy of Education at the Institute of Education University of London, UK.

Exploring Well-being in Schools

A guide to making children's lives more fulfilling

John White

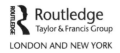
Routledge
Taylor & Francis Group

LONDON AND NEW YORK

This edition published 2011
by Routledge
2 Park Square, Milton Park, Abingdon, Oxon, OX14 4RN

Simultaneously published in the USA and Canada
by Routledge
711 Third Avenue, New York, NY 10017

Routledge is an imprint of the Taylor & Francis Group, an informa business

British Library Cataloguing in Publication Data
A catalogue record for this book is available from the British Library

Library of Congress Cataloging-in-Publication Data
A catalog record has been requested for this book

ISBN13: 978-0-415-60347-8 (hbk)
ISBN13: 978-0-415-60348-5 (pbk)
ISBN13: 089-0-203-81554-0 (ebk)

Typeset in Galliard by
FiSH Books, Enfield

Printed and bound in Great Britain by
TJ International Ltd, Padstow, Cornwall.

For Patricia, Louise, Jamie, Rolf and Bonnie Rae

Contents

Introduction

In 1930, the economist John Maynard Keynes predicted that by 2030, the average standard of living in Britain would have risen eight-fold and there would be a 15-hour working week (Skidelsky, 2009). By then, he thought, people would have turned away from economic goals towards enjoying a fulfilling life.

We are now under twenty years from Keynes's target. The average standard of living is five times greater than in 1930, but working hours are still long. We persist in getting and spending. Keynes's vision of well-being for all seems to have receded far into the distance. Or has it?

Whether or not the millennium made people think of fresh starts, it has been hard not to notice, since 2000, a new preoccupation with a happy life. The media keep returning to it: yesterday's *Guardian Review*, for instance, carried a three-page feature, fronted by a huge clown face, proclaiming that 'the pursuit of happiness is making us miserable'. Schools have made the headlines with happiness lessons. The late Labour government put children's well-being at the heart of its policy for schools and families.

We will not realise Keynes's dream by 2030, but we might just be reconnecting with it. This book is a nudge in that direction. It is about what education can do to speed the arrival of the well-being society.

Schools as we know them can be strange places. A god-fearing science teacher on the radio this morning was telling us how, although he disbelieves in the theory of evolution, he teaches it to his boys so that they can do well in public examinations. I'm less interested here in the religious aspects of this – although I'll be coming back to related matters – than in the implication that schooling is, centrally, about exam success.

We should have left this sad piece of nonsense behind us with the twentieth century. Its schools were caught up in a regime of getting on, doing ever better, getting more and more efficient – but within a system that had lost sight of what it was about. This book presents a new vision. It suggests that schools should be mainly about equipping people to lead a fulfilling life.

In one way, this sounds banal: isn't this what we all expect of them? In another, it is anything but. If we were *really* aiming at fulfilment and had a blank sheet to plan how we went about it, schools, especially secondary schools, would become very different places. As things are, too many are dominated by totems – academic rigour, no-nonsense discipline, hard work, examination star rating, places gained at university. Theirs is a self-justifying enterprise. Examined microscopically, its parts cohere together; but seen as a whole, it lacks a convincing rationale.

I hope to show that making well-being central to the school's life is far from a bland statement of the obvious; the idea is an immensely rich one. If we take it seriously, there are a thousand and one ways in which schools will have to change. I have made a start in setting out what some of these might be.

What we need before all this is clarity. Well-being, fulfilment, flourishing – call it what you will – is at last gaining prominence on the political and educational agenda. But what it is remains murky. For the author of yesterday's *Guardian* article, psychoanalysis is the key to its hidden treasures. For 'Happiness Tsar' economist Richard Layard, it is all to do with pleasurable sensations. Some think that we should not yoke together pleasure and well-being in the first place. Some argue the flourishing life is one where you succeed in getting what you want. Others reject this.

Part of the obscurity comes from philosophical uncertainties like these. But there is more to the book than philosophy. For one thing, fascinating though such discussions are in themselves, *here* they are always harnessed to educational ends. Schools working to the new well-being agenda need a clear picture of what well-being is.

For another thing, we can't ignore the society we live in. This colours how we think and, not least, how schoolchildren come to think about well-being. You would be one tree short of an arboretum if you believed that wealth has no place in this. But how much money do you need? Is failure staring you in the face unless you're rolling in it by the age of 40? The same goes for celebrity. Can you cheerfully pass through life as a nobody?

There are other common beliefs about well-being that need probing. The association, for instance, between well-being and leisure. Was Keynes right to set such store by work reduction? If so, how does this square with the regime of industriousness found in our schools? Are they, indeed, the last redoubts of the Protestant work ethic? Should they be?

How far are the secular heirs of a once-religious world still walking in its shadows? What role does our spiritual, as distinct from our bodily, nature play in our well-being? Is the project of equipping children for this-worldly well-being a gigantic mistake? Should we rather be shaping them into morally good people, able to meet the obligations that God, or some secular counterpart, such as Reason, has imposed on them?

The topic of well-being ramifies into all these questions, tensions, confusions and shadows from our past. I have been touching on these in what may seem like a scattergun approach. A small spider has been spinning away above my computer as I have been spinning out these words beneath it. Like it, I have been scuttling out in this direction and that, returning every so often to a central node, and then speeding off again to make yet more connections.

All these threads are, in fact, linked together, and form a coherent whole in the course of the book. My underlying aim is educational improvement. If we want to base education on well-being, what parents do should be first on our agenda. Good parents have their children's flourishing at heart – not just in the future, but *now*, in the games they play with them, the outings they arrange, the intimacies in which they live together. If being a parent meant compelling one's children to do all sorts of things for which they have little inclination, few would willingly take the job on. Yet this is what their fellow educators in the schools often have to do. If both parties are to work together, who should learn what from whom?

If there is a case for bringing schools closer to families, both could well be more distanced from universities. There is everything to be said for formal learning beyond school; but there is less to be said for the conventional pattern of full-time degree studies at 18 or 19. This enslaves secondary schools to the insistencies of university entrance, with all the perversion of the curriculum, examination stress and spiralling competition for places that we are now beginning to recognise are a major social problem. If we want schools to be seedbeds of human flourishing, there must be some better way.

It is time to be more systematic, so I will describe how the book's argument unfolds. Part 1 looks first at the extraordinary upsurge of interest there has been since the millennium in well-being as a social and educational ideal. Chapters 2–13 explore commonly held accounts of well-being, weigh them against each other and pick out the most promising. The discussion takes teachers, students and parents, step by step, through this landscape, working upwards from the short, easy rambles of its early chapters to more challenging journeys, occasionally with some stiff climbs. Each of the 12 short chapters is divided into two halves. While the first looks at ideas about well-being, the second takes up educational issues that they suggest.

Why do people understand well-being in different ways? The shift from a religious world-view to a largely secular is one reason. Fewer people now believe that personal fulfilment belongs to eternal spirits, and that its prospects are aided by a devout life of hard work and moral rectitude on Earth. More of us now locate it in the life we live as a certain kind of ape. Yet shadows of the religious outlook are still long; witness the persistence of the old work ethic, the way we adulate the achievements of the intellect (AKA 'soul') and uncertainties about whether we should live for others or for ourselves.

Chapters 2 and 3 discuss this religious legacy and its manifestations in education. Schools, especially post-11, are still places of dutiful striving for future rewards, even if those rewards are this side of the grave. The curriculum still keeps pure intellect at the top of its pecking order. In values education, moral goodness wins out every time over personal ends.

In a religious world, what one needs in order to get to heaven may include such things as a pure soul, faith, uprightness, knowledge of the wonders of God's world and good works. Clean drinking water is not on the list, neither is food nor shelter. But most of us, in our very different age, value these and other goods as basic prerequisites of our flourishing, given the kind of animals we are. Chapter 4 looks at what schools can do to teach children about their well-being needs and to develop appropriate dispositions. It also peers ahead into the landscape beyond need satisfaction: what counts as a fulfilling life, assuming your basic needs are broadly met?

I've thought for some time that you can usefully divide people into those who merely watch television and those who also appear on it. Given the extent of regular viewing, it is not surprising that so many in the first group attach such value to being a household face for millions. Close neighbours of celebrity are wealth and so-called 'positional' goods – like fashion items or well-paid jobs, or success in international football matches, which are prized as signs of superior status. In Chapter 5, I examine how far the pursuit of fame, money and positional advantage can contribute to one's well-being. Many of our children are dazzled by these things. Should schools do more to help children see them for what they are?

A life of pleasure-seeking need not go with the pursuit of fame or wealth. The *dolce vita* is a closely related dream ideal of our secular world, one often lambasted from Abrahamic pulpits and by serious-minded journalists. Chapter 6 critically examines Jeremy Bentham's view that pleasure is the key to human flourishing, as recently restated by the economist Richard Layard. Whatever one's verdict about hedonism in general, there at least seems a cast-iron case for making learning enjoyable and not something to be endured for the sake of goods beyond it.

In Chapter 7, we come to one of the most widely held views about what it is to lead a flourishing life. This has to do with success – not 'being a success' in the eyes of the world but getting what one wants out of life as a free, autonomous agent. It is the whole-life version of being an ideal consumer in the economic sphere. Each of these takes for granted a *Which?*-like knowledge of possible options: goods and services in the one case, activities and experiences in the other. On this model, children at school need to be acquainted with a wide range of life options. How encyclopaedic should this provision be?

The chapter also raises doubts about this desire-satisfaction account. Does it matter if what you most want in life is to play slot-machines all day, or to make people afraid of your power, or to want their attention 24/7? What is missing here, according to a different take on well-being, is the notion of *worthwhileness*.

Chapter 8 explores this new perspective. It has radical implications for how we think of schooling. Among other things, it challenges the view that covering the ground is the main task: making sure that no child leaves school without induction into every major branch of knowledge or every major life option. Throwing oneself into one's pursuits, not in a half-hearted way, but, as we say, losing oneself in them, now has a much higher priority. This chapter is the hub of the book. Later ones examine the problems it throws up, as well as practical implications for social and educational reform.

Chapter 9 redeems an earlier promise to look at the place of work in a fulfilling life. The persistence of the work ethic can make it hard to see what this might be. Should we make a clearer-cut distinction than usual between work in which you are more than willing to lose yourself, and work you undertake because you have to? Do schools, as well-defended fortresses of the work ethic, need redesigning in order to become nurseries of well-being? What role should work, both autonomous and heteronomous, now play in them?

Tolstoy's philosophy, following traditional Christian doctrine, was that we should live for others. This seems a world away from the motif of individual fulfilment threaded through this book. It challenges its plea that schools should bend their efforts to the latter. Is naked self-interest all that is left to us once we give up religion? In our new secular age, should schools really be urging children to live for Number One? I try in Chapter 10 to defuse this kind of worry. It rests on an illicit polarisation between personal well-being on the one side and morality on the other. I show how schools do well to think on different lines. They often find themselves in a conceptual fog on the links between moral goodness and personal flourishing, and are not helped by the low priority given to these in the curriculum.

Chapter 8 insists that the activities and relationships that make up a flourishing life must be worthwhile. But how do we tell if something is worthwhile or not? Are there authorities to whom young people and the rest of us can turn? Is there mileage in an appeal to our shared human nature? Chapter 11, in which these and other questions are discussed, is clearly leading us away from the foothills of the earlier chapters. It celebrates the immense proliferation of worthwhile pursuits over the last few centuries and the growth in the number of people with inside experience of them. This leads to unexpected implications for the way we think about citizenship education.

People sometimes say that in a secular world, art is taking the place of religion in helping us to make sense of things – that with its aid we celebrate the bright fleetingness of life rather than dwell on colourless eternity. It is no surprise, therefore, that aesthetic notions help to shape the argument of Chapter 12. This interrogates the claim that some worthwhile pursuits go deeper than others. It is said to be the school's job to provide 'depth' as well as 'breadth'. But how are we to characterise this? Is it to do with specialisation in an academic subject? Is it connected in some way with spiritual development? Do literature and other arts have a role here, in drawing us down from the sensuous surface of life to hidden layers of reflectiveness and feeling?

We come, in the last chapter of Part 1, to what, for some people, is the deepest question of all: What is the meaning of life? But how far should we go along with what looks to be the assumption here that life *has* a meaning? Does this only make sense if there are purposes beyond our natural lives in terms of which they make sense? And if you *don't* believe in such purposes, does that make your life meaningless? Is there a non-religious sense in which we can talk of a meaningful life? Is this the same as a flourishing one? As with many of the issues raised in earlier chapters, those raised in Chapter 13 lend themselves to small- or large-group discussion in schools – and not only in religious education classes.

Part 2 weaves together the threads spun in Part 1 to produce a new vision of what schools should be about. After a brief résumé in Chapter 14 of what well-being involves, Chapter 15 outlines how the wider society would need to change to bring this more within everybody's reach. It points to wide-spread differences in people's life chances and looks to reforms in welfare and work reduction to help iron these out. The chapter concludes with an argument for a remodelled higher education system that, among other things, frees up the later years of secondary schooling for a more fulfilling regime.

This leads us neatly into Chapter 16, the first of two longer, school-orientated chapters centred on every child's flourishing. It asks what priority this should have in the whole panoply of educational aims, not least economy-centred ones. Still in wide-angled mode, it discusses what schools in particular can do to further this vision, building on the person-centred practices of family life. It sees as a first priority setting desirable aims. Yet policy-makers much prefer *not* beginning with aims, but with lists of subjects. We need to get away from this lazy kind of planning and start from a defensible account of well-being goals. Among these, traditional ones to do with the acquisition of knowledge, though important, are subordinate to the personal qualities we all need if we are to enjoy a fulfilling life.

The vision would be incomplete without mentioning learning arrangements. Are 'happiness' lessons a way forward? Should we rethink the balance between activities that children are *compelled* to engage in and those they choose? In Chapter 17, where I raise these questions, I also build on points made in Part 1 about work-based, non-work-based, collaborative and solitary learning. On the way, I make a strong plea for more pupil discussion of issues about well-being picked out in Part 1. A shift towards well-being goals also bears on assessment. How can we get beyond the widely acknowledged inadequacies of conventional testing and examining and rely on more sensible ways of finding out what children are learning?

The book argues for a radical shift of direction in schools policy. It seeks to dissipate the hazy thinking, to which we are all prone, about what should be one of its most deeply embedded values, the child's well-being. The book's message is applicable to school systems across the globe. In every society, including those still emerging from religious shadows, there is massive uncertainty about what constitutes a flourishing human life. Every society is affected by powerful messages in the media about success, wealth, pleasure, fame and getting what one wants. Everywhere, schools are ladders to reach the good things of life, as conventionally understood. Everywhere, some young people make the upper rungs, while millions remain below.

Whether we live in India, China, Nigeria, North America, Europe or elsewhere, this book suggests that we can do better than this. It encourages us to think more clearly about this most fundamental of human values, as the first step in setting our schools on a more appealing path.

My own life has been spent in Britain. It is British fog that I have had to grope my way out of into clearer air – not literally, for the smoke-ridden London of Dickens and Sherlock Holmes is now long past. I am talking about the confused ideas that have been swirling around me for most of my life about what human life is about and what education should be for. It is not surprising that much of the material I use in this book is taken from the society I know best – my own. This applies, not least, to Chapter 1 of the book, where I look at the new drive in the UK since 2000 to improve the well-being of its children. But even the later chapters in the book, whose ideas speak to people more universally, often take their colour and examples from the environment I know best.

Despite this, readers outside the UK will find the arguments accessible and appealing. In some cases, they will be able to translate what I say about how British history has shaped ideas about well-being and education into their own cultural terms. If Britain is now increasingly exercised about what values should guide it in a largely secular age, it is not alone. The shadows that Protestant Christianity still casts on post-religious Britain are paralleled elsewhere by those cast by Muslim, Judaic and other faiths.

It is time for the whole world to detach itself from an educational paradigm that has got us in its grip and rethink what education should be, centrally, about. In China, as we heard in Britain, many children are becoming unhealthily fat because they have lessons that can last until 8 o'clock in the evening, with homework to follow and no time for exercise. As in Japan, Malaysia, Brazil, Britain and elsewhere, they are having to keep their heads down over their science, mathematics, languages and geography textbooks so as to maximise their chances of a place at a good university, a well-paid job and a nice house. Every year, the competition increases and the bar rises a notch higher. The more this continues, the less joyful will young lives become, both for those on the fast track and for those worsted by the competition.

We need, across the world, to stand back. Is this really what schools should be about? Is this insane competitiveness our only option? This book suggests that it is not.

Part 1

Well-being and education, step by step

Chapter 1

Children's well-being in the new millennium

The new millennium has brought a new focus in the UK on children's well-being. Not, of course, that schools and other agencies had nothing to do with this before 2000; but the last decade has seen a step change.

Three developments in the educational world have been:

- The *Every Child Matters* agenda. Launched in 2003, this is about improving the well-being of all young people from birth to age 19. In 2007 it became a key plank of government policy in the shape of the *Children's Plan* for England and Wales. Part of this policy has been about what schools, in particular, can do.
- Before 1999, maintained schools in England and Wales had no nationally prescribed aims to guide them. From that year, an extensive list of these was included in the *National Curriculum Handbook for Teachers in England* (DfEE/QCA, 1999). It states that among the values and purposes that underpin the school curriculum and the work of schools,

    > foremost is a belief in education, at home and at school, as a route to the spiritual, moral, social, cultural, physical and mental development, and thus the well-being, of the individual.

    Since 2007, the aims have been redrafted for secondary schools, but pupil well-being is still prominent. It is most noticeable in the headline aim that all young people be enabled to become '*confident individuals* who are able to lead safe, healthy and fulfilling lives'.
- The third development is about promoting well-being through lessons and programmes specifically devoted to it. The most celebrated example is from Wellington College, an independent school in Berkshire. In 2006, its website announced:

    > This autumn term, students at Wellington will be the first in the world to start regular lessons in well-being (known colloquially as 'happiness').
    >
    > http://www.wellingtoncollege.org.uk/page.aspx?id=595

Within the maintained system, in 2008 a new subject called Personal Wellbeing entered the 11–16 curriculum. Like its sister subject Economic Wellbeing, this is now to be a statutory part of the curriculum.

The recent drive to promote pupils' well-being has been remarkable. Before the millennium, the term 'well-being' scarcely figured in the educational lexicon. A decade later, its use is ubiquitous.

Why this change? It is hard to say. Later historians of education will be better placed than us to make full sense of it. Meanwhile, we have to do the best we can with the pieces of the jigsaw we happen to possess.

The trigger for the *Every Child Matters* initiative was the murder in London of Victoria Climbié and people's consequent awareness that children's services, including education, need to be better co-ordinated around a set of common priorities if such tragedies are to be prevented. These five priorities are that all children should be helped to be healthy, stay safe, enjoy and achieve, make a positive contribution and achieve economic well-being. I will come back to these shortly.

The background to the second development – about well-being as an aim of the curriculum – was growing dissatisfaction with the National Curriculum of 1988. Many thought its intellectualist conception of education, built around traditional subjects, was too narrow. The five *ECM* goals were also grist to their mill.

The appearance of specific lessons in well-being (or happiness), at Wellington College not least, owes a lot to the 'positive psychology' movement inaugurated in 1998 by Martin Seligman in the USA and promoted in Britain by the Cambridge Well-Being Institute. It focuses on the empirical study of factors that make people's lives happier and more meaningful.

Influences from several directions have converged, therefore – from the worlds of social welfare, curriculum reform and academic psychology. All this has happened in the last decade. Why? Is it coincidence, or something indicative of a wider cultural change?

Support for the latter comes from the enormous success of Richard Layard's 2005 book *Happiness: Lessons from a New Science*. Layard, as an economist, adds yet another perspective to the three already mentioned, while also relying on psychology. He touched a chord with the public in his claim that greater wealth does not bring greater happiness. His figures show that since 1950,

> in the United States people are no happier, although living standards have more than doubled... The story is similar in Britain, where happiness has been static since 1975 and (on flimsier evidence) is no higher than in the 1960s. This has happened despite massive increases in real income at every point of the income distribution. A similar story holds in Japan.

(Layard, 2005: 29–31)

It may be that the new interest in well-being that has typified this decade reveals a change in the *zeitgeist* – a feeling that we need as a society to draw breath and refocus on what makes life really worth living. It may be that we are beginning to see the shift of concern – from economic growth to well-being – that Keynes predicted for early this century. If so, whether this is an ephemeral mood or proves to be a historic turning point, must be left to future historians to discuss.

What is this 'well-being' that has now become so salient? Are the various organisations and individuals concerned with it all dealing with the same thing?

The 2008 UK government document *The Role of the School in Promoting Pupil Well-being* defines 'well-being' in terms of

> the five Every Child Matters outcomes that children should be healthy, stay safe, enjoy and achieve, make a positive contribution and enjoy economic well-being.
>
> (DCSF, 2008)

Why should *these five items* be taken to constitute well-being? The first two, health and safety, look more like necessary conditions of it than constituents. If so, why just these two and not other *sine qua nons* like shelter, or law and order? Is it because *Every Child Matters* originated in issues of child protection? If so, has it been sensible for government to rely on the *ECM* scheme in school policies meant to apply not only to abused or neglected children but also to *every* child?

As we have seen, the lessons in well-being at Wellington College are also known, colloquially, as 'happiness lessons'. Is well-being the same as happiness? At a practical level, is well-being something that can be taught in hourly bursts?

And what conception of well-being do we find in the 'positive psychology' that has been so influential at Wellington and elsewhere? Is it true that 'happiness' is divided into three very different realms – the 'pleasant life', the 'engaged life' and the 'meaningful life'? (Seligman *et al.*, 2009: 296). How can one assess how well a person's life is going? Are reported levels of life satisfaction adequate as evidence?

The new school subject, *Personal wellbeing* has three components: 'critical reflection', 'decision-making and managing risk', and 'developing relationships and working with others'. It may seem intuitively likely that these are elements in a flourishing life, but why just these? What is the larger canvas on which they have a place?

Finally, we come to Richard Layard's book, *Happiness*. Is he right in equating well-being with feelings of pleasure? Can one not be flourishing while sweating away at some problem in theoretical physics in the absence of such feelings?

What these questions show, collectively, is a totally blurry picture of what well-being is. They give plenty of attention to this aspect or that – safety, working with others etc. – but how the bits are meant to fit together is unexplained. This is why we have to turn to philosophy. We need to work through the topic trying to find the best account that we can of what well-being is.

Some of the issues just mentioned come up again in the succeeding 12 short chapters of Part 1. In them I explore the idea of personal well-being in more depth, separating its strands, guiding us through its twists and turns and showing how it applies to what does, and should, happen in schools and families. I do this in the belief that teachers, parents and other educators need an accessible, guided tour to the major landmarks. At each stage of the journey (i.e. in the second part of each chapter), I draw breath and ask what the upshot of the argument is, so far, for education.

Chapter 2

Initial questions

We'll each be around, if we're lucky, for 70 years, perhaps more. We want to have a good life, to be happy. How should we go about it?

It's not easy to get a good view of things, especially in the age we live in. There can be fog on the other side of the windscreen and we may have to go carefully until the road gets clearer.

One reason for the obscurity is this. In Britain, as in many other countries, we live in a society that is becoming increasingly secular but has not fully emerged from the religious world in which it has its roots. This is not surprising. When I was a boy, there were bronze pennies in circulation dating from 1860, the year after the publication of Darwin's *Origin of Species*. A post-Darwin world is only a few generations old. The Christian world preceding it had been in place for well over a thousand years. It is not surprising that its influence is still strong today.

Take personal happiness. We all want to lead a happy life. Most of us take it for granted that happiness, if it is to be found anywhere, belongs this side of the grave. But a traditional Christian view has been that blessedness must wait till heaven, for those who make it there, that is; the rest can forget it.

This traditional Christianity has taught us that our mortal life is a preparation only. It has no value in itself. This creates a tension in our thinking. Most of us believe that this life is all we've got. It is only here, if anywhere, that happy lives are made. But this is at odds with the ascetic religious message that if people think that happiness lies in the pleasures of food, drink and sex, exercise, good company, having fun, reading novels, going to the theatre, they are deluded. Living a good life on this Earth is not about being a selfish hedonist; it is doing one's duty before God, living in moral uprightness.

Because of this legacy, many of us, religious or non-religious, are not clear how we should lead our lives. We speak of 'the good life', but in what way should we take this? As a life of fun and enjoyment? Or a life of moral goodness?

How should we live? For ourselves, or for others? Or for both? We have no settled view on this. The religious, or post-religious, voice inside us says that the best life is the saintly one. The ideal, if only we could attain it, is something like a famine relief worker in Africa, a dedicated nurse in a hospice, a Samaritans counsellor. This is a life well spent – even for a secular person who has no thought of an afterlife. 'What are we on this Earth for?' we ask ourselves. And the answer we know already: it is to live for others, to leave the world a better place than we found it, to make some small contribution to reducing the poverty, cruelty, neglect and misery that abounds in it.

Something else within us tells us that 'What are we on this Earth for?' is the wrong question. It assumes we're here for a purpose. But are we? If Darwin is right, life is directionless. We are, each of us, the product of millennia of blind change, of struggle, extinction and survival. The goals and bonds of Christianity neither delight nor frustrate. The earthly happiness it has called illusory is genuine after all. The 'animal pleasures' it has derided are indeed the pleasures of animals – sex, food, drink, play, domination. And what are we but animals? Where can our fulfilment lie except in activities like these?

Life is short. Rosebuds must be gathered. As long as we have vigour, energy, exuberance, we'll give the joys they bring full licence. Priests have called this our 'lower nature', in contrast to our eternal soul. But this is a fairy tale, a nonsense. All we have is a few decades – of youth, maturity and slow decline. Let's make the most of them. Let rooms be filled with song and dancing. Let corks be pulled. Let laughter and loving make our nights too short.

Deeper within there is a different message. This can't be all there is to life. We may be no more than beasts, but some beasts are less beastly than others. What can magpies do but fight and fornicate and scavenge? What can my tom-cat do but hunt, eat, doze in a sunbeam? If we, as human beings, do these things, it is through our own choice, not because we have been programmed to be able to do nothing else. We alone, as far as we know, are aware that we exist. Rabbits can see and hear; mice and starlings can feel pain. Human beings can have these experiences, too, but we alone are conscious that we have them. And this makes all the difference. We are not nature's prisoners. We live and we love – and we reflect on our living and our loving. We have the capacity to rise above our appetites and view them at a distance.

Which means we *do* have a lower nature and a higher one after all. There is a side to us to which the purely biological story fails to do justice. We are all self-conscious creatures, not in the sense that we blush when we're looked at, but in that we – unlike anything else in the universe, to our knowledge – are aware that we are alive, can remember our past, can aim at goals in our future. We not only have relationships with other people; we are also conscious that we do. We are aware that these relationships have pasts and possible futures, that the webs they make and destroy constitute much of what makes life important to us. We not only see and hear, but can also fashion these forms of perception into the arts of painting, poetry and music.

Which of our voices should we listen to? Our Christian background again comes into the picture. We are dealing with two answers to the question 'How should I lead my life?' One looks to our own self-fulfilment, our own happiness; the other looks to what we can do for others. Self-interest versus morality. For a certain sort of Christian, morality is all-important. Our life is built around obligations – to love God, to love our neighbours as ourselves, not to commit adultery, not to lie or covet, to forgive those who trespass against us. Self-concern gets in the way of moral duty. It presents temptations that we must learn to resist. Lust, greed and impatience pull us down towards animality.

It is because morality has been so central in this tradition that we, its secular heirs, have acquired a far clearer idea of what we morally ought to do than of what counts towards our flourishing. We know that we ought to love our children, be kind to our neighbours and help others in distress; that we ought not to lie, hurt people, cheat, steal, kill or break our promises.

By contrast, our notion of personal fulfilment is much more uncertain; and in more than one way. There is no settled view amongst us as to what it consists in. There is also no consensus about what part it should play in our lives in the first place. Isn't a life in which it figures more prominently than in the traditional Christian picture too self-involved, too caught up in the pursuit of self-interest?

Issues for education

This is the first of the *Issues for education* sections in Part 1. Their aim is to flag up educational questions about well-being arising from the main text. A fuller and more systematic treatment comes in Part 2.

I begin large. Should schools and families bring children up to devote their life to moral striving for the sake of a life to come, or see this world as all there is?

In the Britain or America of 1860, most of them would have taken the first line. Few do today. Yet echoes of heaven-centred attitudes are still heard, especially in our slow-to-change school systems. Schools, especially those for older students, are still places of dutiful striving for the sake of future bene-fits. The difference between 1860 is that, for most people, the blessedness in prospect is wholly this-world: the joys of university life, a good job, a nice house, a comfortable existence. *That* is what makes all the hard work one does at school so worthwhile – all that forgoing of pleasures, all that girding oneself up for public examinations. 'Say not the struggle nought availeth . . . '

Others would put the school's contribution to well-being another way. If children are to lead a flourishing life, what they do at school should not merely prepare them for it; it should *embody* it. Learning is apprenticeship. If we want three-year old Conor to grow up into a considerate person, we encourage him to share his diggers and bendy buses with his friends and enjoy cuddling his newly arrived sister. If we want him to lead a fulfilling life, we induct him *now* into fulfilling activities, hoping that, when he goes to school, his teachers will do so too.

Unashamedly, this book follows the apprenticeship model. Later chapters fill this in. It is a complex story, but in this part we tackle it piece by piece, leaving Part 2 to present the overall picture.

Although, like most people, I believe in this-world fulfilment, I am aware that in some religious schools and families the more radical view still persists that education should take the afterlife seriously. Some faith schools that censor books in their libraries for their sexual references, and some homes that ban television for religious reasons, may have little time for promoting personal flourishing as most of us now understand it.

Is a religious school doing the right thing by its students if it presents life on Earth only as a spiritual struggle leading to beatitude elsewhere? Many of us would call this indoctrination. But is it less indoctrinatory to get young people to believe that death is the end of everything?

Indoctrination is keeping minds closed. One way to avoid it is this. We have good reasons for tying well-being to our lives as this-world animals – more telling reasons than for locating it in paradise. These reasons justify us in bringing children up in the former metaphysics rather than the latter. At the same time, they should be encouraged to make up their own minds about the possibility of life after death. Where their well-being is to be located is, after all, of the first importance to how they are to live their lives. They need to discuss both this question and the question on which it depends, about whether there is a divine being.

The revised English secondary school curriculum of 2007 has favoured a move towards 'big ideas' rather than specific items. Yet schools are all but discouraged from discussing one of the biggest ideas of all. The question whether or not God exists is mentioned in the *Religious education* curriculum, but *only* in the explanatory notes – as one example among many of *possible* 'ultimate questions' that schools *might* want to take up. If they do take it up, there is no compulsion on them to examine it from a non-religious perspective, as distinct from a religious one.

It is hard to defend this. We need to insist that all children engage with the question of whether God exists, and in a many-sided, rather than a one-sided, way. The same goes for the issue that depends on this, about where human fulfilment is to be found. What 'bigger ideas' than these could there be?

I am aware that I have not shut down the dispute. Not everyone will agree that we have better reasons for confining well-being to the natural world than for linking it to the supernatural. This book is not the place to marshal all the arguments for this conclusion – although I hope that the case built up through the remaining chapters of Part 1 will do something to support it. For the most part, I shall be taking it for granted that most readers of this book will go along with me – and that among its religious readers there are many as attached as I am to the fulfilments of this world, even if they cleave to more than these.

A central consideration in writing this book is that, emerging as we are out of the shadows of an older, religious world, we have as yet no sharply defined picture of what human well-being is and how this should impact on the work of families and schools. Parents and teachers, like the rest of us, are prey to confusions and uncertainties arising from clashes between the old world and the new. How, if at all, does their remit to bring children up as morally good people mesh with the greater self-centredness that the new emphasis on well-being apparently brings with it?

This and a welter of other questions are explored in the chapters that follow. The next one takes further the theme of the religious legacies – or shadows – that, often unnoticed, have persisted into our more secular age. From Chapter 4 onwards, I begin to put together what I hope is a more clearly defined picture of our well-being and of its educational ramifications.

Chapter 3

Well-being: some religious legacies

1

A familiar move that some religious people make is that the secular world is full of confusion about how we should live and the way out of this is to go back to the certainties of the Bible or the Koran. My own take on this is: 'OK, there's plenty of fog around, but there are better ways of dispersing it. By *thinking*, for instance. By the painstaking separation of strand from tangled strand.'

The main change in western culture over the last few centuries has been the substitution of one world for two. In Christian cosmology, the world in which we live and die is inferior to the divine, eternal world in which, if fortunate, we shall live as immortal souls.

The fog has a lot to do with this dichotomy. For a start, in the two-world story there are already different accounts of well-being: one (a misguided account) for the ordinary world around us, and another (the true story) for the invisible one.

In the ordinary world people are prey to all kinds of temptations because of their animality. They are driven by desires for sex, food, drink, wealth, domination, partiality to themselves and to their group. They think their happiness revolves around things like these. But they are deluded. All these pleasures, if ever they achieve them, end with death. The only true blessedness, for those who reach it, lies in the invisible world.

What shape it takes there is itself more than a bit misty. A story concocted for the masses makes heaven an up-market version of much that attracts us here below – a lot of lolling around, plenty of nectar and ambrosia, and, in some religious fantasies, exclusive access, for men only, to dozens of beautiful virgins.

Another story, the one for the *cognoscenti*, is altogether more cerebral. The core of our being, hidden behind its bodily façade in mortal life, is our eternal soul. Freed from carnal encumbrance, it engages, and can only engage, in spiritual contemplation. Liberated from the body, too, it loses its appearance of separateness from other conscious beings. What once seemed an individual entity participates in the divine consciousness itself.

All this yields two images of personal fulfilment, an illusory one and a real one. Indulgence in bodily pleasures, and pure spiritual activity.

The dichotomy's long shadow lies across our secular age. First, the body. The slightly fusty, male-orientated ideal of 'wine, women and song' has become more alcoholically varied and gender-sensitive, and song has proliferated into all kinds of genres. What was reprehensible in a religious age is now, for many of us, cool. The temptations of the flesh, once reined in by a moral-religious code, are now given all the space they need. And, the new hedonism says, why ever not?

A similar transformation has occurred at a higher-order level. One of the first theories of well-being in the new secular age was Jeremy Bentham's idea that the happy life is one with the greatest balance of pleasurable sensations over painful ones.

Not everyone is happy with this. Bentham's great successor, John Stuart Mill, distanced himself from what he thought some would see as a 'philosophy for swine'. There are higher pleasures as well as lower ones, those of the mind as well as those of the body. People acquainted with both will tell you that the former are superior in quality (Mill, 1861: Ch. 2). If you think sipping a pina colada on a balcony in Tobago is what it is all about, you are plain wrong. You would do better going inside, opening up your laptop and starting your next critical article on Flaubert.

What is this, someone might say, but a secularised version of the two-worlds story? (And remember that John Stuart had a father brought up as a Presbyterian.)

Adulation of the mental, preferably as far removed from bodily associations as possible, is a massive presence in our culture. You will find plenty of *Telegraph* readers and writers lamenting that tourism and media studies are now on the curriculum of some universities. But have you heard similar snipings about mathematics or philosophy? As a philosopher myself, I always enjoy the sudden awe in the faces of those who hear the answer to their question, 'What do you do then?' (It recedes a bit when I state that I am a philosopher of education.)

Among philosophers themselves, the same hierarchy is apparent. Can you imagine political philosophy or aesthetics ever being high up the status ladder? The top spots are only for those most adept at the most abstract – philosophers of language, mind, metaphysics and logic.

Can you imagine wranglers and senior wranglers in sociology as well as in mathematics? Mathematics connotes cleverness, and if you want to discover the cleverest people in England, what better than the Cambridge University practice of ranking its best mathematical undergraduates first, second, third etc.? Francis Galton, who had his heart set on a Wranglership, was shattered not to make it. He consoled himself by exploring in Africa, but still remained attached to mathematics.

This is seen in his comparison of the mathematical ability of a (English) spaniel and a south-west African tribesman, much to the detriment of the latter (Chitty, 2007: 31). When he got back home, he founded the discipline of eugenics, beginning with his classic 1869 study *Hereditary Genius* (Galton, 1978). This claimed that the most intellectually able among us owe their gifts to their heredity. Foremost in the groups he studied were Cambridge Wranglers.

Francis Galton, scion of a famous line of Quakers, but not a Christian himself, illustrates another secular – or perhaps semi-secular – legacy from that creed. I'm thinking of the notion mentioned above about one's loss of individuality when entering the world of eternity and one's consciousness becoming fused with the divine. Galton believed in a scientised, Darwinian version of this. At the end of *Hereditary Genius* he writes:

> ...men and all other living animals are active workers and sharers in a vastly more extended system of cosmic action than any of ourselves, much less of them, can possibly comprehend...they may contribute, more or less unconsciously, to the manifestation of a far higher life than our own, somewhat as – I do not propose to push the metaphor too far – the individual cells of one of the more complex animals contribute to the manifestation of its higher order of personality.
>
> (Galton, 1978: 376)

This scant respect for human individuality – so different from the liberalism of John Stuart Mill – leaves little room for talk of *personal* well-being rather than the flourishing of a larger entity of which each individual is a part. In different forms, the down-rating of the individual was a *leitmotif* of one strand of late nineteenth and early twentieth-century thought. You find it in the eugenicists, including Hitler and the National Socialists; and you often find it in both of Hegel's heirs, the Marxists and the philosophical idealists. On one side, Nature; on the other, Class or State. The Christian God may no longer have been in favour, but his role as an entity in which we can lose our separateness, yet realise our true nature, lived on.

Today, in an age when Christian shadows have grown thinner, there is less enthusiasm – at least for the present – for holistic fantasies. We take the independent existence of the individual more as read. This is why there is so much interest these days in how, in an increasingly secular framework, people can best live their lives.

2.

I have suggested that some of the tangled threads in our thinking about flourishing can be traced back to a more religious age.

• our ambivalent attitude to a hedonistic ideal of life, not knowing quite whether our animality is still to be transcended, or whether it should be celebrated;

- our adulation of abstract thinkers, the Einsteins and Hawkins; and our denigration of hairdressers, gas engineers and 'soft' curriculum options;
- our urge, or what is left of it, to sink our individuality in an entity more significant than ourselves.

Take another issue. Philip Larkin wanted the toad, *work*, no longer to squat on his life. Margaret Thatcher couldn't get enough of it. 'She has never stopped working 19 hours a day,' said her friend Lord Archer in 1995. 'She has nothing else in life. She can't stop, and she doesn't know how to. She starts at 6 am and they have to drag her to bed at night' (Paul Vallely, *The Independent*, 27 May 1995).

What part should work have in the flourishing life? More than one of the six Mitford sisters were horrified when the Second World War came along; not only because teasing, adorable Adolf was no longer available for tea parties, but because war service regulations turned their existence upside-down. They were forced to labour in canteens or bookshops; and almost driven to doing their own housework through a deadly shortage of servants.

Nancy wrote to Jessica (whom she called Susan) in May 1944:

> Susan isn't work dreadful. Oh the happy days when one could lie & look at the ceiling till luncheon time. I feel I shall never be right again until I've had trois mois de chaise longue – & *when* will that be?
>
> (Mosley, 2007: 200)

While the Mitfords were aristocrats, Margaret Thatcher was the daughter of a Wesleyan Methodist grocer. Over two or three centuries, for these and other non-conformists, work had never been a toad. It was willingly sought and pursued as a religious/moral duty. But the point of it was still, in one way, personal fulfilment. Unremitting hard work in the service of God, the success that this brought, the deliberate spurning of a softer, more carnal existence, all stood one in good stead when it came to the judgement whether you would be saved or damned.

How do we think of work today? For most of us it is as much a necessity as it was for the Puritans and their followers. But it's no longer a duty imposed by God.

This brings us to work's role in well-being. It is, for most of us, a basic need. I will be saying more in Chapter 4 about basic needs in general, but what about the area of life that comes into view once basic needs are satisfied – the region where friendship, binge-drinking, reading Betjeman, trekking across Bolivia, playing computer games, gardening, showing off one's tattoos, and astronomy all claim to be elements in a fulfilled life? Is work to be counted among these elements? It's hard to say. Working in atrocious conditions in a

Welsh slate mine is one thing; working as a highly respected portrait painter another. And what about Mr Don't-mess-with-me, the super-hood who works nearly as hard as Margaret Thatcher and loves every minute of it?

We will come back to this in Chapter 9. I have been talking about our religious heritage, especially in its non-conformist reaches. For devout religionists of earlier times, relentless hard work was a normal feature of life – indeed, its central feature. It dominates *our* lives, too. But while the religionists had no doubt that work is an ingredient in the good life, we are far more confused about this.

This is partly due to the ambiguity in the term 'the good life', already mentioned. When the old believers talked of the good life, they meant a life of moral goodness, one spent in obedience to God's laws. On this definition, work was, for them, unquestionably part of the good life. Whether it is also a feature of a personally fulfilling life here on Earth – a 'good life' in *that* sense – is not a question they would have asked.

Issues for education

Since 2007, the subjects in the National Curriculum regulations for England and Wales have been listed alphabetically. Before then, they were presented like this:

> English, Mathematics, Science, Design and technology, Information and communication technology, History, Geography, Modern foreign languages, Art and design, Music, Physical education, Citizenship, Personal, social and health education.

Despite the change, the pecking order of the old list persists. English, maths and science are still the 'core', tested subjects. Not far below them come other knowledge-rich areas like history, geography and foreign languages. The direction still goes from 'harder', more academic, more abstract subjects, down to what many people see as more peripheral ones.

From the perspective of a fulfilling personal life, it is odd that subjects to do with the arts and with our personal and social life are mainly at the bottom of the heap. In our day-to-day life, not all of us need a knowledge of algebra, geometry, chemical equations and medieval history. But *everybody* has a personal, social and civic life. And while few adults turn to maths as a source of personal fulfilment, enjoyment of the arts is universal.

Cultural history throws light on this. It is well known that puritanical beliefs have played a large part in British life over the past four centuries, as they have in America. Fainter echoes of Matthew Arnold's diatribe against non-conformist narrow-mindedness in *Culture and Anarchy* were heard in reactions to Margaret Thatcher's call for a return to 'Victorian values' a century later.

Today's National Curriculum has its roots in this tradition. We see the same depreciation of the arts in favour of the transmission of theoretical knowledge, the more abstract the better. There was once a plausible rationale for this; and, interestingly, it had personal flourishing at its heart.

The radical Protestant tradition had no time for the classics-focused education that had been the norm before the seventeenth century. Guided by thinkers like Jan Comenius, its schools and academies prepared young people not only for worldly success but also for their eternal life as pure intellects. As creatures made in the image of an omniscient God, their duty was to amass as much knowledge as they could about the divinely created world.

Among the subjects they learned, the most abstract disciplines – logic, mathematics and physical science – had a special place. Part of their appeal was their very abstractness. A person about to shed the things of this world for eternal life had no use for the perceptual delights of the arts, for emotional subtleties or for anything else anchored in the bodily organism. Pure logical thinking was a different matter. Mathematics, the basis of the new physics, existed in a world detached from empirical constraints. It fitted the bill well. Centuries later, the educationalist Fred Clarke (1923: 2) could still write that 'the ultimate reason for teaching Long Division to little Johnny is that he is an immortal soul'.

Acquiring knowledge for its own sake, and abstract knowledge in particular, has long enjoyed a privileged place in the fulfilled life. Originally, this was life in heaven, but there are still echoes in our own more secular world and educational system. We adulate 'brains of Britain' and 'masterminds', as well as infant Mensa members of IQ 160 who are dab hands at number series. On the educational status ladder, we put theoretical knowledge several rungs above practical. In public examinations, we test literature for knowledge of plot and characterisation more than for aesthetic and emotional impact. We still award 'the life of the mind' the winning rosette, and leave the more practical lives that most of us lead as also-rans.

The Protestant legacy also includes a penchant for knuckling dutifully down to hard work. In British society in general, this is less evident now than it was among the Victorian middle classes. Yet it is still the prime virtue of the model British pupil. Schools, especially secondary schools, are the main surviving stronghold of the Protestant work ethic. They may not go so far as John Wesley did in 1749, when he said of his newly founded Kingswood School that 'we do not allow any time for play on any day'. And they may not quite follow Wesley's packed curriculum, for six-year-olds upwards, of Reading, Writing, Arithmetic, English, French, Latin, Greek, Hebrew; History, Geography, Chronology; Rhetoric, Logic, Ethics, Geometry, Algebra, Physics, Music (Wesley, 1749: 2). But the legacy to us of unremitting diligence is plain enough.

If we want schools to do more to promote pupils' well-being, is it time to rethink this? Industriousness, after all, is not necessarily a good thing. It can be a dark quality, as the regime of any of Stalin's or Hitler's labour camps testifies. *Self-chosen*, rather than constrained, work is a different matter. Dickens and Trollope drove themselves hard as writers, but they did so out of commitment. Most of the hard work we expect of pupils is in subject matter they are *obliged* to study. From the standpoint of their own welfare, how helpful is this? Does it matter if much of what they study leaves them cold?

There are further questions. Do we send children to school to work or to learn? Is there a difference between the two? Does all school work produce learning? Can children learn things without engaging in work? If so, and if schools are primarily about learning, should they make more space for non-work activities? We look at these and other issues in Chapter 9.

From the next chapter onwards, I turn away from religious legacies and build up an account of well-being from independent foundations. But before I do so, one last thought. In the religious age from which we have now all but emerged, your own salvation was of central importance. It mattered more than anything else in the world that you were on the road to heaven rather than hell. Hard work at the vocation to which God had called you, making use of your God-given gifts and talents, would lead you to a successful career and to general acknowledgement that you belonged to his elect.

This has cast shadows into our more secular times. We may not urge children to toil away at their homework and their exams so that they will be saved, but we do still want them to have a 'good job' and the comforts that go with it. We may have divested the terms 'calling', 'vocation', 'gift' and 'talent' of their theological meaning, but we still run 'gifted and talented' programmes to identify those most likely to succeed.

Remember, too, that in the religious age only *some* would be saved. These days we may not talk about an 'elect', but we do use the term 'elite'. It carries the similar implication that not all will be members of it. And this way of thinking has coloured the way we organise our schools. So much of twentieth-century, and now twenty-first century, British educational policy has been about creating privileged spaces where some children – with rich parents, a high IQ, selected as 'gifted and talented', or who work the hardest – are given what is seen as a better education than others.

As we shall see, our secular pictures of what it is to flourish in life are bound up with elitist ideas about 'doing well'. This creates a problem if we want *everyone* to lead a fulfilling life.

Chapter 4

Well-being and need satisfaction

It seems we can agree on one thing at least: if personal fulfilment is to have any place in our life at all, we all have certain basic needs that must be satisfied for it to be possible. That human beings require oxygen in order to live is a scientific fact. That they need food and drink is undeniable. Clothing and housing are minimally more controversial. Some human beings in hot parts of the world can go without clothes, but for others of us it is, again, an objective truth that we need them to survive. Is the same true of a dwelling-place? Perhaps many of us could live some kind of hand-to-mouth existence without one. If basic needs are for *bare survival*, housing is less copper-bottomed a candidate than food.

But our topic is not bare survival; it is having a flourishing life in a modern society like our own. What do we basically need for *that*? Housing immediately passes the test. What *kind* of housing we need – whether a bed-sit will suffice, or nothing short of a four-bedroomed villa – is a further question. But at least we can agree on the more general point that we need somewhere to live. The same is true elsewhere. We all need a minimum of good health in order to flourish, even though our lives might hang on by a thread without it. How *much* good health we need is moot. Some of us would like to go on to 90; others prefer a shorter and merrier life. A rotting liver or lung is the last thing most of us want, but for some people the pleasures of drinking and smoking might make it worth the risk.

What else should be included as a basic need? Income, obviously; but how much? Can we flourish on a pittance? Or do we need a hefty lump of disposable income? A good education seems another obvious candidate. But there's massive disagreement about what it should consist in. Personal liberty – freedom of speech and action – is also indispensable in a modern democratic society. As with income and education, there will be differences of opinion about what this entails in detail. But there's little dispute that, in some shape or other, we all need it along with all the other goods if we are to thrive.

All these items fall within the purview of government. It does not necessarily provide them itself. But it at least provides a regulatory framework of minimum standards. It is not for nothing that we talk of a 'welfare state'.

Luck is also a basic need. Whatever shape our life takes, we all need good fortune if we are to flourish. A plane crash, a natural catastrophe, an unprovoked assault, a breakdown in health or a stock market crash can bring us personal disaster. Nothing can eliminate bad luck completely. Government, as well as such institutions as private insurance, can do something via welfare policies to make up for it, but nothing can rule it out for certain.

If all our basic needs are met, do we thereby lead a fulfilling life? Hardly. I could be well off, healthy, well-educated and generally blessed with good luck, but find myself in a job where I'm bored out of my mind, or in a relationship likely to turn both parties into depressives. We need to go beyond the basics. They provide, after all, only the necessary conditions for a thriving existence. What it *is* to thrive is still in question.

This brings us back to the radical differences of opinion about this topic mentioned earlier. Here are some of the issues waiting to be discussed:

1. *Pleasure.* Whether or not I seemed more than usually glum when I last went to my barber, he said, *a propos* of a dying woman in a drama on his shop TV, 'We're all going to die, aren't we? Enjoy yourself! You live in a big house? Sell it, get a small one. Use the money. Go on holidays. Stay in hotels. Enjoy the time you have.' He fixed me so insistently in the eye as he was saying this that I felt this was a message especially intended for me, something he felt he just had to tell me. But perhaps it wasn't.

    What role does pleasure play in personal well-being? Should we fill our lives with it? Could we manage without it?

2. *Work.* When I walked away from the barbers, feeling an exhilarating coldness on my scalp, I wondered if his hedonistic message was more about his own circumstances than mine. Did it reflect his own dreams? As he lay back on his leather sofa watching women dying on his overhead monitor as he waited for a customer, was he half in Barbados, sipping cocktails by his five-star pool?

    For most of us, work occupies most of our days. Our short, unique post-Darwin existence is more than half filled with it. What contribution does it make to our flourishing? Is it something we would rather dream ourselves out of? Or can its role be more fulfilling?

3. *Look at me.* You couldn't miss the number-plate on the Merc that curled in front of me into the last space in the gym car park: 'POL1CY'.

    Not the most personal of messages, I agree, not like 'T1 AMO', but, even so, unmissable.

    If you've got money to burn, why not flaunt it? Let people see you're not a nobody. Tell them about the view over the river from your apartment in your gated ex-warehouse complex. Tell them about its pool, its bars, its cinema. Or if you are a bit lower down the status ladder, why not send everyone you know the 72 pictures of your recent cruise? Both of you grinning from your deckchairs, kayaking, snorkelling with the dolphins?

4. *A child's-eye view.* A recent survey of ten-year-olds asked them 'What is the best thing in the world?' The top spot was 'money and getting rich', beating the usual favourite, 'being famous', into second place. What place does fame have among the constituents of well-being?

5. *How would we know?* How, in any case, does one find out what these constituents are? Is there some objective way of ruling some things in and others out? With some basic goods, there is, as we saw, no problem. It's an objective fact that we all need food and drink. But once we get beyond the basics, are we still on such firm ground? Can we say that a primary school child who only wants to be famous is on the wrong track? If so, why?

Or is what counts as well-being much more up to the individual? Suppose you want, above all, to be rich, or to enjoy family life, or run your own company, or spend your free time surfing, or reading Persian literature. And suppose you succeed in doing what you want to do; is this to say that you are thriving? Is well-being a matter of fulfilling your deepest desires *whatever* these may be – even if what you most want is to be the highest-scoring serial killer there has ever been? We come back to the big question already touched on. How does our own well-being relate to the world of moral obligations?

Issues for education

The five topics just sketched all prompt questions about children's learning – about, for instance, what attitudes they should acquire towards the pleasure-seeking life, towards fame, wealth and work. Since I deal with all these curtain-raisers in later chapters, I concentrate here on the prerequisites of a flourishing life, whatever we say in the end about the shape it might take.

Traditionally, pupils' basic needs have not figured in schools' programmes. These have rescued children from ignorance about academic matters and have equipped them with basic skills, but have had little room for anything more personal. My own secondary schooling is an example. The only basic need remotely connected with its curriculum was physical exercise. But the compulsory rugger, cricket and gym that made up my physical education were not part of a programme to promote personal well-being. They had more to do with dutiful attachment to the manly virtues. As for sex education, this was wholly off the radar – unless you count learning about the mating habits of the earthworm. I envy the wholly beneficent personalised learning about masturbation that a friend of mine received at 13 in his bathroom from an older cousin. A school lesson or two, suitably adjusted, but with the same reassuring message, could have saved me and many others from years of inner turbulence.

These days things have moved on. Since the arrival in England of the very traditional National Curriculum in 1988, more and more prescriptions to do with meeting learners' basic needs have been added to it – about health education, including drugs and sex education, regulating one's emotions, staying safe, having a balanced diet and money management.

From the point of view of education for well-being, these accretions are welcome. True, they have, as often as not, been reactions to some perceived catastrophe in the making: the high rate of teenage pregnancies, drug addiction among the young, gang and knife culture, childhood obesity. Rather than gluing new bits onto an already packed school curriculum, it might be better to step back a bit and think in a more measured and many-sided way about what the school should do about basic needs.

Its role overlaps with that of the family. This is one area among many where, if we are indeed taking well-being more seriously, the two major providers will have to work more closely together. In an educational context, basic needs divide into two groups. Take sewerage and sensible eating. Both are health-related, but while families and, increasingly, schools can do a lot to develop the latter, providing the former lies outside their remit.

On the one hand, then, there are things beyond the school's control, like clean air, water, power, housing, a police force, banks, government, and on the other, things in which it can play a part, like the proper regulation of bodily desires (e.g. for food, drink, sleep, elimination, exercise, sex) and emotions (e.g. fear, anger, joy, compassion), keeping free from bodily damage (e.g. tooth decay, physical attack, reckless activity, alcohol and other drug abuse) and managing money.

Let's home in on this second category. The task of families and schools is to build up appropriate dispositions in all these areas. The job is many-sided. Take the desire for food. Parents, reinforced later by teachers, have to shape children's habits, so that they come to eat the right things on the right occasions and in the right way. At first this is largely a matter of behavioural training. Three-year-old Fintan learns not to keep asking for another Colin the Caterpillar sweet, not to push his uneaten baked beans onto the table, but to see mealtimes as occasions for enjoyable social interaction. As his understanding grows, he is better able to grasp the reasons his carers give him for these things. He learns more in time – and here schools come to share the responsibility – about why some foods are better for his health than others, about distress he may cause to others by unsuitable behaviour, and a host of other things. He learns to be appropriately flexible in his eating habits, seeing it, perhaps, as all right to stuff himself at parties, but not at other times. Gradually, he comes to see the larger point of all the food management into which he has been initiated. He connects it, perhaps at some less-than-conscious level, with similar dispositions he has been acquiring in the areas of exercise, emotional control, keeping safe, etc. He comes to see the point of all these things as good for him, as necessary elements in his own flourishing.

The pattern of upbringing in all the other second-category areas is the same. The aim is disposition-shaping. Parents and teachers are helping the child to become a certain kind of person. As far as schools are concerned, this shifts the emphasis from their traditional role as purveyors of knowledge. Hence, for instance, the irritation that the new (at time of writing) British Minister of Education, Michael Gove, expresses when he says, 'In making schools institutions which seek to cure every social ill and inculcate every possible worthwhile virtue we are losing sight of the core purpose, and unique value, of education.'

To reject Gove's stance is not to deny that schools have a responsibility to pass on knowledge in this area. They deepen the work that parents have begun in developing children's understanding of different foods, the effect of exercise, what things are dangerous, personal budgeting, and so on. They bring to bear relevant knowledge from medical science and chemistry, social studies and other fields. The knowledge they transmit has, on this view of education, a purpose outside itself. It is an integral element in building up desirable dispositions.

With basic needs in the first category – like sewerage, transport and the police, over which schools have no jurisdiction – their task, again building on what parents do, is different. It is to enlarge children's understanding of these things, not now as a part of disposition-building but in order to give them a wider picture of what they need as requisites of their flourishing – and not just their own. A basic needs education extends into what we *all* require. Eating sensibly and having good housing and a decent transport system are important not just for me, but for all of us. Although the way each of us enjoys a fulfilling life may be very different, one person leaning more to the arts, another to extreme sports or family activities, we all have the same fundamental needs. This is hardly surprising, seeing the kind of animals we are and the kind of society in which we live together. Part of basic needs education is to bring children to appreciate this commonality. It touches, at its more philosophical end, on issues of what it is to be human, and how, in the light of this, we should conduct our common life.

It also requires the acquisition of a large amount of knowledge, including historical knowledge – about medicine, housing, government, the food industry, the international drugs trade, banking. It is hard to see where the list would end. Mr Gove and his fellow traditionalists need not worry; the person-centred upbringing I have been outlining is far from antipathetic to the transmission of knowledge. It demands it.

The discussion has not covered all basic needs. Take freedom. In order to lead a flourishing life, at least in our kind of society, we *choose* the activities we engage in. We are not forced, dragooned, compelled to do them. I am far from saying that no school lessons should be compulsory, but if the government really wants to enhance pupils' well-being it should insist on their freely choosing many of their activities. Schools could learn from families on this. Parents and grandparents know how vital it is to let children freely get on with activities in which they are fully absorbed – and how counter-productive it often is to try to get them to do things they really don't want to do.

Receiving an education is itself a basic need. Schools not only help to provide it at the first-order level, but at the second-order level also they can and should encourage reflection on education's place in human well-being, on what it should contain and on how the education system has come to be what it is.

These are some of the ingredients of basic needs education. I come back to the topic in Part 2 as part of its synoptic account of education for well-being more generally.

Chapter 5

Fame, wealth and positional goods

1.

Let's come back to those ten-year-olds from the last chapter. You will remember they were asked 'What is the best thing in the world?' 'Money and getting rich' was their most popular answer, with the previous year's favourite, 'being famous', dropping to second place. 'God' came in at number ten, just below 'nice food'.

The top two goods often go together, and not only in the minds of children. I'll come back to getting rich, but let's now concentrate on fame.

It's no surprise that young children rate this highly. They are exposed to it every day on television. But are they right to do so?

Is being famous a *sine qua non* of a flourishing life? If it is, this radically cuts down most people's chance of having one. Or is it merely something that might make one's life go better, a desirable addition to it for some people if not essential for everyone?

What is fame anyway? It has to do with being well known in circles much wider than intimate or face-to-face relationships. In the ten-year-olds' answers to 'Who is the world's most famous person?', the Manchester United footballer Wayne Rooney came second. Not surprisingly, perhaps, given his extraordinary skill and the global adoration of Man U. (On the latter, a Chinese friend of mine was among the student protesters on Tienanmen Square, Beijing, in 1989. He was down for security duties on the Square on the day of the massacre, but was officially excused so that he could stay at home to see his favourite team in a cup final.)

Wayne Rooney did better than Jesus at number three. As for the most famous person of all, that had, of course, to be God – despite being separated by Wayne from himself as his son!

Fame does not have to be worldwide. Dr Crippen is famous in Britain but not, I imagine, in Angola. Vic Usher, a prominent local politician in the London Borough of Barnet council in the 1980s, is now immortalised in the street named Victor's Way. This may sound like a boulevard in a post-1945 Soviet metropolis, but, in fact, it skirts the car park near the McDonald's on

Barnet High Street. Vic was famous enough in his day in the more politically sensitive reaches of his own borough, but how many, even in neighbouring Camden, Brent and Enfield, had ever heard of him?

Vic reminds us, too, that fame can be as hemmed in as much by time as by space. God has had an amazing run for his money to date, and, timewise, Caligula and Genghis Khan have both done creditably. Vic's short-lived success is now extinguished, probably for eternity.

Were our ten-year-olds right to esteem 'being famous' so highly? Towards the end of his book, *The Third Reich*, Michael Burleigh (2000) writes:

> Concern with posterity was apparent enough among the Nazi leadership, whose final weeks were akin to rehearsals for a drama, designed to perpetuate their malignant presence into indefinite posterity, an endeavour in which they have been notably successful, judging by their all-pervasive presence at the start of the new millennium. (p. 788)

Burleigh goes on to describe Goebbels's vision of a film they will be showing in 100 years' time, 'a fine and elevating' picture of 'the terrible times we are living through'. A few days later, he is reminding Hitler that:

> If the Führer were to meet an honourable death in Berlin, with Europe falling to the Bolsheviks, within five years at the latest, the Führer would become a legendary personality and National Socialism mythic, because he would have been sanctified by his greatest and last act . . . ' (pp. 790–1)

Is *any* kind of fame a good thing, even that of a deranged mass-murderer? We can surmise, from God and Wayne, that the children had something more positive in mind. The 'fame' they prized may well be shorthand for 'being well-known for doing or being something desirable'.

This definition means we can leave on one side not only the Crippens and Caligulas, but also those who get into the limelight for having done something quite pointless – a streaker at a rugby match, for instance, whose only motive is to get attention.

However, the streaker is on every television newscast that day. Next morning her rather nice body is in every newspaper. Isn't that an achievement in itself? Who says it's pointless? (And why do I remember, all these years later, that her name was Erica? Doesn't that underline her success?)

Restricting fame to what's desirable may not help that much. For who is to say what's desirable? For you it may be things like listening to cello recitals or breeding Irish terriers. For the streaker it is getting noticed by as many people as possible. And once we've got to this point, why not bring evil-doers back into the frame? The Nazi leadership, for instance?

All this brings us back to the *leitmotif* of the book. What is a flourishing life? Once basic needs are met, what kinds of experiences count towards it?

Which count against? Do we keep in playing with our children and keep out streaking? If so, why?

Or is personal well-being to do with realising one's desires, *whatever these may be* – even exhibiting one's body to a mass public?

It's a hard question and I will come back to it. Meanwhile, let's look at things that everyone would accept as desirable – being an extraordinarily gifted footballer, a major poet, the discoverer of DNA. Why, if at all, is it a good thing to want to be famous for things like these?

Quite often, fame *happens* to people although they don't seek it. A poet works away at her craft. Her whole attention is on making her work as perfect as possible. She gets noticed, is the leading poet of her generation, is talked and written about everywhere.

Would the ten-year-olds do better to undergo the discipline of becoming an athlete, an engineer or an actor and leave aside their dreams about celebrity? On this view, if fame comes along in the wake of their achievements, fine. If it doesn't, also fine. What matters is engaging in the activity, doing it as well as one can.

Or would the children do even better for themselves by desiring fame *as well*? If so, what are the benefits? If they succeed in their wishes and become celebrities, that might make them richer. Fame can bring extrinsic rewards; but that makes it replaceable by other things, like a legacy from a wealthy uncle. Does it have any intrinsic benefits? How desirable is fame in itself?

A life is a stretch of time. How well we fare has to do with how well we spend our minutes, hours and days. The children, say, are training hard to become athletes or actors. If, in addition, they are after fame, how does this colour how they spend their time? They spend much of it *thinking what it would be like* if they were a celebrity. They linger over what others would think and feel about them, how they themselves would react to all the adulation.

A similar story can be told about those who *have* made it, who *are* celebrities. Many of them still desire fame in the sense that they want to hang on to or expand the fame they have. How might this affect how they spend their time? Here again it is likely to involve a lot of thinking, not only and not particularly in the sense of reasoning things out, but also all sorts of other dreamier empathisings and wonderings. They put themselves in the place of all the TV viewers who saw them in the charity show last night, vicariously feeling the watchers' admiration and envy. They think how much their parents would be proud of them if they were still alive.

Time spent wanting and enjoying fame is time spent on activities like these. How worthwhile are they? If worthwhileness has to do with enjoyment, this kind of thinking can certainly be very pleasurable. But not always. A well-known person can be put out by a waspish review or a photo with the wrong profile. Fame can bring pain as well as pleasure – and not only as a result of one's imaginings. Think of begging letters and paparazzi.

Even when the thoughts are wholly pleasurable, if all you want is to have nice images in which you are the central figure, you can get these from ordinary daydreaming. They don't have to be associated with fame. So there must be some better reason for wanting celebrity than pleasurable thoughts alone. It must have to do with the specific pleasure that comes from thinking that many people are admiring you.

But why should this be *valuable* as well as enjoyable? What if you are massively deceived? You think you are loved, but in fact most people hate you. You think they envy you, but in fact they see you as pathetic. Is the pleasure you feel worth having?

Are people sensible, then, to want to be famous? If they succeed, they may be in line for extrinsic rewards, since fame can bring money, power and other things in its train. A further question concerns what the relationship is between these rewards and their well-being. I'll come back to it in the next section. As for any *intrinsic* benefits, it is not at all clear, given the doubts just expressed, what these might be.

Even if there *are* intrinsic benefits, how likely is anyone to get them? Seeing that few can become famous, any particular person's chance of success is slim. How many suburban minstrels are there, I wonder, who, from time to time, get down their guitar from the top of the wardrobe and see themselves on stage facing a waving forest of arms?

2.

Better than fame, at the moment, is money and getting rich. At least that's what our ten-year-olds thought. For them it is the best thing in the world.

Are they right? If we're talking about basic needs, income is obviously one of them; not just enough to survive, or even to get by, but enough to thrive.

But the children in the survey were not into basic goods but into the best things in the world. How far is getting rich among these? We don't know if the children meant this as an end in itself or not. If it *is* just an end in itself, not prized for the goods it can buy, the envy it creates, or any other external good, it is hard to see what is desirable about it.

I was walking down a side street in west London today and passed a large shop window. Through it I could see several women sitting next to each other and wiggling their bare feet in glass tanks full of miniscule darting fish. The price per half hour of this piscatorial foot spa was as much as some who live in east rather than west London earn in a day.

People often want great wealth and what it can buy partly as a sign of superior social standing. They want them because few can have them. They are examples of what Fred Hirsch (1977) was the first to call a 'positional good'.

It's deafening in Cannes these days, they say, because of all the helicopters taking off from and landing at their private pads. Below the super-rich, the merely wealthy belabour each other with the latest improvements to their place in the Lot or their 'little lunch' at the Ritz hotel. Even the rest of us go for goods we kid ourselves only few can have, as when we buy car insurance puffed by a celebrity. A management post is positional if you want it because it singles you out from others; likewise academic achievements – as expressed, for instance, in the triumphal old student song to the tune of the Red Flag 'The working class can kiss my arse, I've got my PhD at last'.

How valuable is it to possess a positional good? I mean possess it *as* a positional good – bearing in mind that a winter holiday in South Africa can be sought for intrinsic interest as well as status-marking. Is it good for you just because it is something you very much want and now you have it?

The answer may not be clear. Suppose you own an £18 million Picasso, whose aesthetic merits mean nothing to you. Does the benefit lie in pleasurable thoughts about the thousands who see your name beside it when you loan it to the Met? Does it matter if they think you a self-important philistine or never notice the name of the lender? Does truth matter as long as you are bathed in comfortable thoughts?

The value to yourself of a positional good is hard to assess for another reason. You may want others to feel inferior to you because they can't afford a personalised number-plate or private education. But even if you want the latter because it is good for your children and without any trace of *schadenfreude*, this may well be at the cost of others' well-being. The more energy devoted to the accumulation of positional goods like wealth and others dependent on it, the more these scarce commodities are likely to gravitate to the few, leaving less for the rest of us. Not all these goods may be worth possessing – the eye-catching car number, perhaps – but income, health and education are basic needs for everybody, and if money, superior medical care and schooling are siphoned off to the few, the many will lose out.

Desiring wealth and other things as positional goods is hard to dissociate from deleterious effects on other people, intended or not. What implications, if any, does this have for personal well-being?

Can my well-being be promoted if I know the goals I seek are likely to make things worse for others? Or does it imply that I must care about their interests?

This is another topic too big to handle now. I will come back to it in Chapter 9 when I look at the relationship between personal well-being and morality.

One last comment on positional goods. All those so far mentioned have been goods sought or possessed by *individuals*. But they can also belong to larger groups, like football teams or nations. If Man U wins the cup, others can't. At the beginning of the World Cup in 2010, the streets of London were a-flutter with English flags. Politicians want top British universities to be among the best in the world.

A question we should ask ourselves more often is: How far does identification with larger groups like these help individuals to live more fulfillingly? Does the promotion of such identification by the media and by politicians intentionally or unintentionally divert people's attention from more certain sources of well-being closer to hand?

Issues for education

The last chapter called for a more many-sided approach to basic needs education. At its more philosophical end, children gain a better-focused picture of the place of basic needs in human life. As I said earlier, 'big ideas' has now become a curriculum planners' buzzword: they want learners to see a wood as well as trees. Chapter 2 suggested more work on whether there is a God. That's a fair-sized forest. Basic needs is another.

Children also have to make sense of what lies *beyond* the prerequisites – to understand what they are prerequisites *for*. This is the first of a series of chapters that explore this.

What is a flourishing life? Powerful forces in our culture put celebrity and wealth at its pinnacle. As we have seen, primary school children soon pick up this message. This is not surprising. When I was young, television was unknown. Radio was a poor medium for glitz, glamour, hype, climactic talent shows, hero worship in sports, interviews in Caribbean mansions. Today, via TV, magazines, the internet and other media, these things are inescapable. Together, they transmit the thought that the good things in life are competitive, for the very few, the talented, beautiful and rich. This chapter has already begun to challenge this, and the rest of Part 1 will cast yet more doubt on it.

If we want children to acquire a more balanced understanding of the good life, we need to do more to prevent them from being daily re-engulfed by this cultural tsunami. But what? Restraining the media raises issues of press freedom and paternalistic intrusion into the choices of autonomous adults. Parents could sometimes do more, by not allowing their children too much exposure to *Britain's Got Talent* and *Heat* magazine; or by involving them in discussions on ethical issues like those raised earlier in the chapter, as well as on the business background to the celebrity cult.

There is a problem where, as so often, parents themselves are caught up in this cult. Does this call for more education of parents themselves, perhaps partly via some of the very media that are generating the problem?

What might schools do? The issues raised by the culture of celebrity and wealth are ideal for class discussion. How appealing is the competitive approach to life that this brings with it? How much would you mind if you went through life a 'nobody'? Is the fashionable attack on the celebrity cult overblown? What is your attitude to those kinds of goods whose value lies in the fact that only few can possess them? What examples of 'positional' goods have you come across in your own lives? How far are people's lives made better by identifying with their sports team or their country in national and international competitions?

These kinds of question, as well as those discussed in the first part of this chapter, could be material not only for discussion but also for role play and imaginative projects woven round them. There is nothing specifically on the pursuit of celebrity or wealth in the two new subjects of the English secondary school curriculum, *Personal wellbeing* and *Economic wellbeing and financial capability*, although the former does prescribe that pupils should be able to 'reflect critically on their own and others' values'. This gives teachers plenty of scope to deal with matters like the one in question – and, indeed, with all the 'issues for education' discussed in this second part of the book.

One way into the topic of celebrity might be via the work schools do in the area of recognition and attention. Of these two, attention is the wider concept. In giving Hazel recognition for her good answer or for her helpfulness, the teacher is also giving her attention. But recognition and attention come apart when, on another occasion, she is sorting out a commotion at the back of the room. Attention? Yes, and in spades. Recognition? No.

Teachers have varied ways of dealing with attention-, including recognition-, seekers. But recognition is important even when, as with Hazel, it is not sought. Teachers show in countless subtle ways how they value children for themselves, as well as for what they say and do; and how they expect them to give the same recognition to others in the school community. They can build on this by making pupils more explicitly aware of the significance of reciprocal recognition in civilised life. There is a helpful overlap here with the work on basic prerequisites discussed in the last chapter, for how could anyone flourish if what they say or do, or, at the extreme, even their very presence, is always ignored or denigrated?

The desire for fame, except when it is notoriety, brings with it a yearning for attention and recognition on a wider scale, and sometimes, as with the cult of celebrity, on a massively wider one. Teachers can build on children's everyday experience to make connections with its larger-scale forms. This includes experience of the pursuit of recognition – harmless enough when Zoë wants a classroom visitor to admire the picture she has been painting, but dubious in far needier instances. How far is desiring fame a yet more extreme version of this?

A related discussion topic is being successful. How important do pupils think it is to end up as one of life's winners, rather than a loser? Does their school reinforce this dichotomy by positions in class, and by the recognition it gives to those who do well in public examinations? How, in any case, do the students conceive of winning and losing in this context? Can one only be a success in life if one gets into a really well-paid job and enjoys the lifestyle this brings with it? If some people end up successful, does this mean others have to be failures? Could we imagine a society in which everybody, barring ill luck, is successful in their relationships and in the work and non-work activities they whole-heartedly undertake, even though few of them live in big houses and have wealth to burn?

The British Council has useful material on success and fame, including a lesson plan and worksheets, at

http://www.teachingenglish.org.uk/try/lesson-plans/success-fame

It is intended for teachers of English as a second language to older students, but may be adaptable for more general use with secondary pupils. A tailor-made plan for a double lesson for Year 9 pupils on the media and self-image is available at

http://www.becal.net/lc/re_pshe_ce/citizenship/yr9media.htm

This also focuses on success, failure and celebrity.

Chapter 6

A life of pleasure

1.

I am aware that I keep putting difficult topics on ice. Three in particular:

(a) the hedonist view that well-being is to be understood in terms of pleasurable experiences and absence of painful ones;
(b) the desire-satisfaction view, that whether or not you are flourishing is a matter of how far you succeed in satisfying your desires;
(c) the relationship between well-being and morality.

I will look at (b) in Chapter 7 and (c) in Chapter 10. But first I'll say something about pleasure, picking up from points in Chapter 3 about our religious legacy. Over the last two centuries, for many of us, Christianity has been turned on its head. What had been the only true reality – the soul's blissful life in heaven – has now become illusion. What had been deceptive – enjoying the one life we have – is the only actuality.

What is it to enjoy this one life? We are animals, sharing many of our characteristics with other mammals. What is the good life for a domestic cat? What is it for Zeus, my tom, to have a fulfilling existence? He is healthy, fed regularly, free to catflap between house and garden as he will, to watch blackbirds from hides among the flowers, slumber in the sunshine and have sex in the moonlight.

Our own well-being, too, is rooted in our biology. As cultural beings, we enjoy more sophisticated pleasures than our pets. We not only have dwelling-places; we furnish them and adorn them. We do more than eat and drink; we delight in cooking, in dining, trying new foods. Our senses of sight and hearing, coupled with our self-awareness, create all kinds of aesthetic delights, while our in-born curiosity, developed by culture, takes us into complex forms of understanding. We can choose among our pleasures, plan for them, enjoy them again in memory. As a scientifically advanced society, we have learnt how to minimise the physical distress that corroded human flourishing in the past – the pains of hunger, cold and disease.

This is an attractive way of thinking. It is not surprising that, when secular perspectives on the good life began to appear in the late eighteenth century, the first and most influential of these, Jeremy Bentham's, was broadly on these lines. Fulfilment lies, he told us, in a life as full as possible of pleasurable experiences and as free as possible from painful ones.

It is also not surprising that the views of Bentham and his utilitarian followers were indebted to the religious world they thought they were leaving behind. They took over as real the life of earthly enjoyments that Christianity rejected as myth. They also took from this religion its moralism – its insistence that our task on this Earth is not to live for ourselves but to fulfil our moral obligations. The supreme moral principle for the utilitarian was, and is, that one should try to bring about the greatest happiness for the greatest number. True, this principle is no longer based on the will of God; it is thoroughly secular. Yet if one tries to live by it, it can be every bit as rigorous as a religious ethic. After all, one's own happiness counts only as one unit among millions. If everyone's interests have equal weight, one's own happiness cannot count for very much.

Bentham's ideas – on well-being as pleasurable experience and on our moral duty to promote the greatest happiness – have shot into the British headlines in the past few years. This is because they have been adopted – and indeed scarcely adapted – by the so-called 'Happiness Tsar', the economist Professor Richard Layard, who, since his creation as a Labour peer in 2000, has been able to build his happiness agenda into government policy under both Blair and Brown. In his book *Happiness: Lessons from a New Science* Layard (2005) tells us that:

> Happiness is feeling good, and misery is feeling bad. At every moment we feel somewhere between wonderful and half-dead, and that feeling can now be measured by asking people or by monitoring their brains. (p. 6)

Using such measurements to assess how happy we are in the UK and the USA, Layard shows, as we saw in Chapter 1, that although incomes have vastly increased over the last 50 years, we are no happier now than in 1950. He presses us to rethink what a better society would look like, concluding that:

> We desperately need a concept of the common good. I can think of no nobler goal than to pursue the greatest happiness of all – each person counting. This goal put us on an equal footing with our neighbours, which is where we should be, while it also gives a proper weight to our own interest... (p. 234)

I will come back to this moral message when I look more squarely in Chapter 10 at how our own well-being maps onto moral demands on us. For the moment, let's stick to whether well-being itself can be understood in terms of pleasurable experiences.

There is certainly something attractive about this suggestion. Depression is on the increase. Lows apart, so many of our days are vanilla-flavoured in mood. We carry on through our tasks in a neutral, fairly joyless, slightly anxious way. Wouldn't it be better for us if we could be lifted? We know that Prozac can help depression and that alcohol and other drugs can change our moods for the merrier. I am not talking about being sky-high 24/7, and agree that addiction needs to be avoided if it has dangerous consequences. But what about something short of that – a greater tolerance of mood-changing substances, so that we felt somewhat happier for somewhat more of the time? Would this not be a contribution to human well-being?

In *Brave New World*, Aldous Huxley outlined a dystopia in which people from the subject class are conditioned to take a happiness pill whenever they feel low. But what exactly is wrong with Brave New World? Is it the pill-taking? Or the manipulation of a lower class by a higher?

We can filter out the political side by imagining a society in which people are not pressurised to stay in a happy mood but do so voluntarily. If we are not easy about substance abuse, we can also forget pill-taking and think of other kinds of mood raisers. The one I have always liked best – not that I have tried it, since the example is as fanciful as Huxley's *soma* – is the experience machine. This is plugged directly into the pleasure centres of the brain and gives you, on demand, the feelings you would be having if you were actually lying on a beach in the Seychelles, walking through young spring woodland or making astounding love. Suppose we could all have sessions for several hours a day on our own experience machine, would this not help the cause of human flourishing?

Some would say we are already in such a world. Multi-channel television is an experience machine in our living rooms. If we add to this all the other instant happiness inducers and painkillers we have in our society – alcohol and Panadol, coca-pods and i-pods, Sea Breeze and DVDs – are we not well on the way to this secular heaven?

2.

It's a sad admission, I know, but I like doing crosswords. Not the quick kind, not the fiendish, but the cryptic sort. I have feelings of moderate pleasure whenever I solve a clue. But most of the time it's a battle to see if I can get into the distorted mind of the setter. More often than not, I can't – and remain frustrated. A.J. Ayer, the philosopher, may always have been able to complete his *Telegraph* puzzle on the bus to University College London, but I usually have to give up on my *Guardian* one.

In terms of discrete experiences, doing crosswords gives me an abundance of negative feelings and too few happy ones; yet I do enjoy doing them.

This seems to knock a wedge between enjoyment and feelings of happiness. Other things do, too. Sitting in a philosophy seminar, for instance, listening to a complex paper, trying both to understand it and to see where its weak points are. This is a world away from watching *Strictly Come Dancing*. Concentration of this sort is painful. You have to grit your teeth to do it. That may be why photographs of famous philosophers are often so grim-looking, all tautness and frowns. It may be why whenever a director of the institute where I work used to meet me in the tearoom, he would say, drawing from Dr Johnson, 'How's the philosophy, then? Cheerfulness keeps breaking in?'

Yet philosophers enjoy their seminars, their writing, their reading of texts, however taxing and painful these may be. Would they have more fulfilling lives if they did less philosophy and had more fun on the beach?

All this creates a problem for the Benthamite view. Enjoyment seems to be coming apart from pleasurable feelings. A world-class marathon runner may enjoy her race despite the endless miles of pain, a judge in a harrowing case of multiple murder may enjoy dispensing justice. Many of those frowning philosophers in the photographs lead happy-enough lives. They have plenty of time to do the things they want – write, read, review, meet, teach, critique. If you made them retire at 40 and promise never again to read Plato, nothing could make them more wretched.

Happy or enjoyable lives are not necessarily to be understood in terms of happy *feelings*. Feelings are things that happen to you and are usually short-lived. When we talk about people enjoying tussling with sudoku puzzles, or cycling in the Tour de France, or helping a needlephobe to overcome her fears, we are not referring to any pleasurable experiences they may have, if indeed they have any at all; we are talking about their being caught up in an *activity* that they really like, and which they pursue with enthusiasm.

Does this suggest a new direction in our search for what constitutes human fulfilment? Should we be looking at agency rather than passivity? Should the spotlight be on the activities that go to make up a human life rather than on isolated experiences?

But Bentham, as the champion of pleasurable sensations, isn't finished yet. He might willingly agree that activities come into the story. People play golf, have drinks with their friends, throw frisbies across the sand. Of course human beings are active creatures, just like tom-cats, but what makes their lives worthwhile is the pleasure they experience in holing a long putt, the feeling of *bonhomie* that a second pint brings, the high that a runner feels crossing the line in record time.

I will leave you to decide whether you think this reply is adequate. Does it account for the enjoyment we can get from activities more painful than pleasant?

Suppose you *don't* think it's adequate and are inclined to think that flourishing is more about enjoyable activity than enjoyable feelings. Here's a question for you. Do just *any* kind of enjoyable activities count? What about the sadistic enjoyment a stasi interrogator got from interrogating people in the DDR times? Did this make his life more fulfilling? Or the enjoyment an addict gets from playing fruit machines day in day out? Would a lifetime of such gratification add up to a life of well-being?

Forget theories for the moment and think of people you know whose lives have gone well for them – or badly.

Laura always wanted to become a doctor. She went to medical school, worked in a hospital for a spell, and is now a general practitioner in a group clinic, married and expecting her second child. When people ring up at 8.30 for appointments that day at her surgery, more than half of them ask to see her as their first choice.

Trevor was a brilliant and much-respected physics teacher in a secondary school for 20 years. But he developed a manic depressive illness so severe that he had to stop work in his forties. The drugs he was given damaged his brain and destroyed his previously impressive powers of thinking. He now lives on his own, with carers coming in to attend to his needs. He enjoys watching videos, especially adaptations of Jane Austen, which he sees over and over again. He also spends part of his time happily 'writing' a new book on science – which turns out to consist in copying from a textbook. He once had a number of close friends, but now few of them visit him, and that infrequently.

Laura's is a flourishing life. Trevor's was, but is now massively diminished. I don't know much about their feeling states or more generally how enjoyable their lives have been, but I am pretty confident about these judgements on their well-being. Why is this?

It seems to have to do with success, with getting what you want. Laura is realising her desires to become a doctor and start a family. There was a time when Trevor was equally fortunate. He had good friends and an interesting job. He would still like to be someone who enlightens people about science, but although in his own eyes he is making headway, in reality he is deluded. He would still like to see more of his friends, but they rarely appear.

Issues for education

Education in pleasure begins with pleasurable sensations, those of taste, being touched, stroked, hugged, tickled, bathed, exercising one's limbs. Young children learn to seek out such feelings, not only to enjoy them when they occur. They ask for cuddles, try to seduce their grandparents into giving them another jammy dodger, want to roll again and again down a grassy slope.

Their sensation-seeking is typically a part of something else – slaking hunger or thirst, or social interaction, or an enjoyable activity. Sometimes it is more atomic. Children want sweets even when not hungry.

Parents and other carers help them to build up appropriate dispositions related to sensation-seeking. This has partly to do with the basic-needs education discussed in Chapter 4. In eating and drinking behaviour, they try to bring their children to want to live healthily. In emotional education, they wean children away from enjoying any thrill they may feel when causing pain or distress to others. Sometimes, though, inappropriate sensation-seeking can take a hold. Young people can turn into bullies, addicts of nicotine, alcohol, other drugs.

What can parents and teachers do beyond encouraging children in good habits? There is work to do in the sphere of the imagination. Some young people's visions of the ideal life are crowded with images of themselves enjoying sunshine, exotic food and drink, admiration, recognition, sex in plenty. These may or may not be linked with the images of celebrity and wealth discussed in the last chapter. Like those, the media generate them in abundance. Teachers and parents can involve young people in discussing the adequacy of such visions. Can a string of passive pleasures like these add up to a satisfying life? How much does it matter if we do not enjoy them in actuality, but only in our thoughts? How far is it a good thing to live in the virtual worlds of television, film, video and magazines?

Teachers can also use literature, film and other arts to stimulate debate about this kind of pleasure. There is no shortage of visual material they can use as triggers. As we have seen, the conscious target of Aldous Huxley's *Brave New World* is a Benthamite dystopia in which even the slightest hint of a melancholy thought is dissipated by swallowing a pleasure drug. Arguably, its relevance is even greater to our own antidepressant-rich age than it was to that of the early thirties when it first appeared.

Students will not get very far in discussing the lotus-eating life without experience of alternatives. We will see something more of these in later chapters. We have already come across a possible confusion that might hamper their thinking. 'A pleasurable life' can mean more than a life crammed with pleasant feelings. When we take pleasure in a conversation, we are not necessarily experiencing shudders of delight or even milder sensations. To take pleasure in an activity is to *enjoy* it, even though, as we saw earlier, this does not have to be a fun pursuit, but could be some knotty theoretical or practical task. Taught in the right way and with appropriate illustrations, most older students should be able to appreciate something of the difference between the *sensation* sense and the *activity* sense of 'pleasure'.

From classroom discussion to educational policy more broadly. Making sure that children's time at school is enjoyable has not always been a top priority. Traditionally, this has been the acquisition of knowledge. How many pupils, like myself when young, simply imbibe, in an emotionally neutral way, what their teachers require them to imbibe, believing in some unreflective way that the school knows best what is good for them?

I was reminded of this recently when I came across a remark by the later

Archbishop of Canterbury, Thomas Secker, about his studies at Tewkesbury dissenting academy in the early eighteenth century. He wrote, 'I apply myself with what diligence I can to every thing that is the subject of our lectures, without preferring one subject before another' (Bennett, 1830: 224).

In Secker's academy, there was a good reason for adopting this attitude. Acquiring knowledge, as we saw in Chapter 3, was a religious obligation. Learners were not meant to throw themselves whole-heartedly into this or that part of their programme, only to cast away as much of the sin of ignorance within them as lay in their power. Today's schools rarely share this kind of religious perspective, but here and there may still retain something of the flat, joyless atmosphere of an earlier time.

A secondary school regime of timetabled slots of 50 minutes each – already known in the academies of Secker's time – may not be the surest way to make each lesson a pleasurable experience. Teachers are trained to seek out hooks to grab learners' attention. But for many pupils, this may do little to allay the dull monotony of it all. The diligent among us mind less. A profile of the new (at time of writing) Schools Minister, Nick Gibb, reports him as saying, about the grammar school he attended, 'What was good about it was that it was rigorous. Every lesson was rigorous, even things like music: it was taught in the same way as chemistry' (*Education Guardian,* May 18, 2010).

Children not so Secker-like may be less enthusiastic. Some of the kids who cannot wait for the end of the school day, and whoop out into the streets when it comes, may be the same young men and women, a few years later, who lay drunken waste to city centres after the end of a boring week at work.

Schools could, and sometimes do, provide a very different kind of cultural apprenticeship. A flourishing human life, as these chapters in Part 1 are beginning to reveal, is one filled with enjoyable and worthwhile relationships and activities, at home and at work. In a country like Britain, we have some way to go in making this a reality for everyone. But in our post-millennial age, in which well-being is rising fast up the political agenda, there is room for optimism. On the way to this more equitable society, and as an initiation into it, we can aim at making every school day an enjoyable experience for every child.

Chapter 7

Getting what we want

1.

All this suggests we need a different account of personal well-being from the pleasurable feelings account – one that has to do with satisfying desires. You flourish more the more you are able to do the things you want to do; you flourish less the less you succeed.

This is an appealing idea, for more than one reason. It copes, I'm pleased to say, with my grim fellow philosophers. They may not climb too many peaks of joy in their professional lives, but they do have a clear idea of what they want – to have a better understanding of thorny problems about the freedom of the will or the body–mind relationship. And they do succeed in satisfying this desire: their understanding deepens with the years.

The desire-satisfaction view can also cope with the attractiveness of the feelings account. Many young people enjoy the bodily pleasures of sports, dancing, sex, listening to loud music, eating and drinking. They go for these partly because they like the sensations they bring with them. They get a buzz from these things. A fogey might deny that any of this is good for them, but the fogey could be plain wrong. The desire-satisfaction view can easily cope with this. What the youngsters want is precisely to get these buzzes, *to experience these sensations.* Insofar as they succeed, they thrive.

Personal fulfilment, then, is getting what you want. A life has been vastly more thriving than another if its possessor has satisfied most of his desires while the other has met with constant frustrations and failed to overcome them.

Like the pleasure account, this version of the good life is one that many will warm to. It fits the tenor of our times. Inhabitants of affluent societies like our own *do* judge the success or otherwise of their lives by this yardstick. If they are reasonably well off, the world is, if not their oyster, at least their green-lipped mussel. They can move into a bigger flat, eat out, cook for their friends, buy a plasma TV, go sun-seeking in the tropics. If people realise their ambitions and their dreams – even if it means going through the pain of doing philosophy – they lead a fulfilled life.

True? My mother, who died a few years ago at 89, was a dedicated smoker all her life. She once reckoned up that since the age of 14 she had got through three quarters of a million cigarettes. She wanted cigarettes every day of her life; and she got what she wanted. If the desire-satisfaction view is sound, this must have contributed to her well-being. Did it, though? People can want things that are not good for them, so satisfying their wants may make their lives worse, not better.

I suppose I should tell you that my mother never inhaled and was never affected by lung cancer. Perhaps the habit helped her to cope with her slightly anxious disposition. This complicates the picture, but the point I'm driving at should be clear enough. There are plenty of drinkers and smokers and users out there whose addictions *are* a threat to their health and overall flourishing.

Many of these want to give up. They both want a smoke or a fix; and also they want to give up. So their wants are contradictory. They pull in opposite directions. This creates another problem for the desire-satisfaction view. How can satisfying want A contribute to your flourishing if it contradicts satisfying want B, which also does so?

Is there a way out? For those who want to kick their habit, A and B are not on a par. Wanting to give up is more important to them than wanting to smoke. It is the same with other things. A teacher who easily loses his temper when his class plays up wants to let off steam, but in a cooler moment prefers to be the sort of person who better manages his anger.

In each of our desire economies, some wants are more important than others. This is true not only of overcoming bad habits, temptations and addictions. As I have confessed, I enjoy doing crosswords. But this does not count for much among my priorities. There are a lot of things that trump it. If I had to choose between doing no more crosswords in my life and never again walking in the country, or writing philosophy, or being with my family, it is clear what would have to go.

This suggests that the desire-satisfaction account needs to be modified. It is too general as it stands and needs refining. We need to restrict the desires in question to those that have some importance in the agent's life, perhaps those that he or she would not willingly give up.

But would this restriction be enough? Take someone who really likes salty foods of all kinds and can't bear the thought of not eating them. At the same time she knows nothing of the health risks she is incurring, especially because, again unknown to herself, she has very high blood pressure and could well be heading for a stroke or heart attack. Eating salty food is bad for her despite its high priority in her life.

This suggests that we need to add something to the desire-satisfaction account about *knowledge*. Getting what you want is only good for you if your desire is well-informed. You have to know what it involves, what the consequences would be of satisfying it.

I often meet an elderly neighbour of ours in the local newsagents buying lottery tickets for the weekend draw. It's a high point in her week, she tells me. Each Saturday she is convinced she is going to win, even though she has only ever won twice, and then only the lowest prize on each occasion.

Is playing the lottery good for her? It does not seem to be. If she knew the colossal odds against her landing a major prize, this might make her see that it's a mug's game and lead her to spend her money elsewhere. On the other hand, it might not. Like a lot of people, she might know the odds are stacked against her, but still enjoy her flutter. The ritual of buying the tickets and watching the coloured balls drop out of the whirling drum is a fixed point in her week. It keeps her going. Her desire is both a well-informed one and also occupies a high place in her scheme of things. So would satisfying it be good for her?

It is hard to see on what grounds you could deny this. Doing so smacks of paternalism. *You* may well think it's a waste of her money, but this is only to prioritise your values over hers. She has her eyes open and knows about her chances. *She* is the authority on what is important to her, not you.

The revised desire-satisfaction view insists that the desires be both personally significant and also based on relevant information. The revision is attractive. It reflects what a lot of people think. It fits the kind of society we live in – a modern liberal democracy. The Benthamite notion, in terms of pleasurable feelings, also fitted the culture of its time. Two hundred years ago, Christian thinking was still dominant. It is understandable that the first major ethical theory that broke loose from it should share some of its assumptions – its thin account, for instance, about this-world happiness. Times have moved on. We now live in a democratic society, one in which nearly all adults are treated – theoretically, at least – as autonomous persons. They are not blind followers of authority, but can participate on equal terms in political decision-making. In their private lives they are able to live as they prefer, as long as they do not prevent others from doing the same. Among other things, they can spend their money how they wish. A free market in goods and services gives them plenty of options from which to choose.

The desire-satisfaction account fits this culture. The individual is the final authority on what constitutes his or her well-being, given the provisos already discussed. It is not surprising that economic theorists have picked up this idea. A market economy needs justification. It has to be shown that it serves the general good, not only the interests of shareholders. The most compelling way of doing this is to point to its role in promoting people's well-being. What is good for individuals includes what satisfies their desires as sovereign consumers, given that they are fully informed about the goods and services they are buying.

The new definition of well-being may fit the culture, but will it do? Perhaps the culture is adrift and needs reorientation. Who can say? Certainly, we should not take over the definition just like that. It stands in need of justification. It is not self-evidently true.

Many of us live by this ideal, at least implicitly. We see our happiness in terms of success in meeting our preferred goals. We understand these to be goals that mean a lot to us, not our preference for butterhead over lamb's lettuce, or one type of pizza over another. (A flyer from Domino's Pizza has just come through my letterbox. It asks, 'With over 66 million combinations to choose from . . . how do you take yours?'.) We accept that we need clearsightedness about our goals so we are not deceived. If we marry, we go into this with our eyes open to pros and cons, are not romantically deluded. In buying a car or a new kitchen, we go off to the library and photocopy the relevant pages of *Which*?

Suppose there is empirical evidence that 80 per cent of the population now lives by this ideal. Would that count as evidence in its favour? It seems to show that it fits the kind of creatures we are. It suits our nature. No one is forcing us to live in this way; we do so very willingly.

But couldn't we, in principle at least, be wrong? Couldn't we be self-deluded? In any case, even if it is true that the overwhelming majority of us lives by this notion of happiness, what does this show? Only that we *believe* this is where our happiness lies, not that the belief is well founded. For it to be so, moreover, it is hard to see how empirical evidence – of whatever sort – can clinch it. For what has to be justified is an *ethical* claim – that the life in which our major informed desires are met is *better* for us, personally speaking, than one where they are not. How can social statistics show what is good or bad?

But where could an alternative vision of the good life come from? It is all very well showing there is space for it in principle; but what can fill the space?

Whatever form the vision might take, it would have to deny the individual's sovereignty over what counts towards his or her flourishing. This seems to mean that someone else may be in a better position to know this. But how could that be? The claim looks like a throwback to a more paternalistic and authoritarian age. If, as a reflective, informed person, I let it be known that my good consists in living in harmony with my gay partner, honing my drumming skills and writing erotic verse, what moralist, priest or presbyter can gainsay me?

2.

We have reached a crux. Do individuals know best what is good for them? Or might someone else know this better than they do? If so, who could this be? And what arguments could be used to support their superiority?

In Chapter 4 we looked at basic needs – the needs that have to be met if we are to lead a flourishing life, like oxygen, food, clothing, shelter, income, upbringing. This is one area at least where individuals are *not* authorities on what is good for them. For many of these basic needs, there is objective evidence that, for creatures like ourselves, survival, let alone flourishing, is impossible unless they are satisfied. This is based on incontrovertible facts about human nature. If we were made of tin – lungless, stomachless, skinless – clean air, food and clothing would not figure among our needs.

But in the last three chapters we have been exploring the territory beyond basic needs, examining what fulfilment consists in, given that our needs are broadly met. Are individuals the final authorities *here*?

If the informed desire-satisfaction view is right, they must be. Once their basic needs are provided for, individuals have the last word on what counts as personal fulfilment in their own case.

It is hard to see how this could be challenged. If some other agency professes to be in a better position than me to tell me how to lead my life, this does look like paternalism. Personal counsellors are becoming a bigger feature now of British life, as they have been in American life for decades. But a good counsellor does not tell you what ends you should follow. They take the ends you have and suggest more suitable means.

Just what is wrong with paternalism? If someone else *really* knows what goals are good for me, perhaps nothing. But how can anyone else have that knowledge? The danger of paternalism is that one party imposes their own view of how life should be lived on someone else. It is not that they have a hotline to the truth that others lack; it is that they are pressurising or forcing other people to do their bidding. Paternalists are close cousins of the abductor. They are kidnappers of the mind.

Paternalism contravenes the first premise of a liberal democratic society, that with few exceptions each adult is an autonomous chooser. If we accept democracy, we accept the informed desire account of the good that accompanies it.

Or so it seems. But is this last claim true? *Does* democracy entail the informed desire view? We have not shown this. Autonomous choice may not be limitless. It may, for all we know, be within certain constraints.

The term 'constraints' provokes a liberal shiver. It seems to point towards a constrainer. But this may be a misconception. Let's agree that in a democracy people should be free to live as they wish as long as they are not harming others. In this sense they live without constraints. No one is preventing them from doing what they want. But they could still be living in a way that does nothing for their flourishing. People are free to live in dirty, unhealthy conditions, or to smoke 50 a day, or never to get out of bed. Liberty and well-being are not the same thing.

I have to be careful. You may think I'm begging the question against the desire-satisfaction account in these examples. Assuming the people know full well what they are doing, why should we say that living in filth or staying in bed all the time are not in their interests? After all, they have knowingly chosen these things. So how come they are not worthwhile, at least for them?

Let me try something different. Suppose there were some way of showing that not everything goes, flourishing-wise. Suppose, just for the sake of argument, the pursuit of truth, beauty and goodness is the one and only key to the fulfilled life. Let's also assume, for the sake of argument, that there are excellent grounds for this position. It would follow that someone preferring above all to lie around all day in bed, doing nothing, would not be on track for fulfilment. But he could still be *free* to live like this. No one need be frog-marching him to the library or art gallery.

I have raised the possibility that what contributes to personal flourishing is not a subjective matter. It is not to do with what an individual happens to prefer, but is more solidly rooted. Admittedly, I have done nothing yet to *show* this. On the way, I've tried to show that being free to do what you want is not necessarily the same as doing what is good for you.

I hear you telling me to cut the cackle. If there are objective values that trump individual preferences, let's have them. If you can't produce them, let's stick with the sovereign chooser.

Let's see what I can do. If there are no limits to what an informed individual may choose, this lets in not only bed-wallowers but also people we can dream up in our imagination who lead very bizarre lives. The sand counter, for instance. This is someone whose main and almost only joy in life is counting the grains of sand on British beaches. You ask him why he does it and he tells you, 'I don't know, it's just great. I can't think of anything I'd like to do more'. You tell him it's pointless, he'll never reach the end and so on – and he replies, 'I just love it'. You talk about all the other things he might be doing, how he is missing out on music, being with his friends, intellectual studies. But he replies that he has a couple of degrees, has tasted all sorts of other activities and relationships, but has always come back to this one passion.

What are we to make of him? He is not mentally disturbed. He can always give a rational response to your questions. He is not counting the grains with some scientific hypothesis in mind. He is a thoroughly informed chooser, able to satisfy his most cherished preference. How can he not be leading a flourishing life?

There are two ways of looking at this. First, as a reduction to the absurd. In other words, the case fits all the criteria, but no one could possibly call this a flourishing existence. The criteria must be wrong. Fulfilment cannot depend so radically on what individuals prefer.

The other way is to dig one's heels in. If there were such a person, there is every reason why sand-counting *would* be in his best interests. The chances of anyone living like this are remote, so it is not a real issue. But the idea that individuals know best what is good for them is still unscathed.

How can we adjudicate between the two positions? A feature of the second is that its reasons give out at a critical point. *Why* is a person's well-being to be identified with the satisfaction of his or her informed preferences? No grounds have been provided. Why, then, should we go along with the idea?

It is certainly deeply entrenched in the culture. Our consumer economy bolsters it with every TV commercial; the press and media reinforce it at every turn. But the fact that an idea has powerful backers does not make it right.

A sand-counter would be leading a massively impoverished life, not a flourishing one. To have done nothing with one's life beyond having counted 673,589,246 grains on Bournemouth beach is to have failed in it. The 'achievement' may get you into the record books, but Guinness is not necessarily good for you.

If we reject the individual's untrumpability, the big question remains: What is missing from the sand-counter's life?

Issues for education

Suppose the informed, autonomous individual is the final authority on what his or her well-being consists in. What sort of education might that point to? One, perhaps, where learners know about a large range of life options from which to choose – and where parents, schools or policy-makers do not restrict them in line with their own preferences, for that would be paternalistic.

This suggests a broad curriculum. If choosing a career, for example, learners have to know something about what different jobs involve. The same goes for choice of housing, friends, holidays, religious affiliations, free-time pursuits: if they are to make sensible decisions, it helps to have some understanding of available alternatives. This ties in with the point made above about the desire-satisfaction account of well-being, that the desires must be *informed* ones.

Would something broadly based, like the English National Curriculum, fit the bill? People often argue for this kind of curriculum – or one akin to it, based on a comprehensive list of 'areas of experience' or 'forms of knowledge' – as providing a 'basis of choice' about what way of life to follow.

I don't know how far Michael Gove, the current Coalition's Secretary of State for Education, would accept the desire-satisfaction account of well-being. He certainly puts great weight on autonomous choice of a way of life:

> Perhaps I value education so much because it has given me so much – but what it has given me most is the chance to shape my own destiny. For generations of my family before me, life was a matter of dealing with the choices others made, living by a pattern others set. I, and those members of my generation who were given the gift of knowledge by wonderful teachers, have been given the precious freedom to follow their own path.

His curriculum preference is for one that is 'traditional, academic, fact-rich, knowledge-centred, subject-based'. Something like the current National

Curriculum, in fact, with a focus on English, mathematics, science, modern languages and other fact-rich subjects like history.

But is this too quick? In Chapter 3 we saw some problems with this traditional answer. Why should we think that a curriculum now long in the tooth, built for the more tradition-directed society from which Gove himself has been freed, should be our best way of promoting autonomous well-being? I am not saying that knowledge of science or history cannot help. Of course, this can help to expand our range of choices, both of possible careers and leisure interests, as well as deepen our understanding of the society in which we are choosers. But other areas of knowledge, not part of the traditional canon, and anathema to people like Gove, can also help in these directions: media studies and sociology for instance.

We can press this further. Take choice of career. Like many young people from an ordinary background, their noses kept to the academic grindstone during their formative years, I emerged with next to no knowledge of the possible careers open to me. Should my schooling have made me aware of what it would be like, and what I would need, to become a financial consultant, a barrister, a civil engineer, a journalist, a landscape designer or a civil servant? Children from more privileged homes may pick up information about these things by the way, but do the rest of us need something more systematic built into our curriculum – something more wide-ranging and emancipatory than conventional 'careers education'?

More generally, how far should the understanding of possible life options – not only to do with careers – extend? In principle, it could fill every minute of every school day. There is so much that children could possibly learn about – all the innumerable jobs they could do, the myriad potential leisure activities, the belief systems they could adopt, the personal and social relationships they could enter into, the human psychology that lies behind these ...

There is also, seemingly, a good reason why their understanding of life options should be compulsory and comprehensive. Unless made aware, in a non-negotiable way, of all the different ways in which they may live, they may miss out on something that could have transformed their prospects. It seems as if nothing less than encyclopaedic provision will do.

Hold on! Would that be a sensible way of preparing children for a fulfilling life? Education is not only about mapping out possible lives ahead; it is also about giving learners plenty of experience of what it is to live flourishingly by inducting them into fulfilling pursuits themselves.

A student could, in principle, acquire knowledge about life options in a Secker-like way, grinding through all the alternatives without any particular enthusiasm. Students need, from an early age, to spend hours of their time whole-heartedly involved in pursuits that they enjoy. As part of wanting them to flourish in *this* world, rather than in another eternal one, we should help them to find fulfilment *now*, while they are children, and not only as an adult.

We face a conflict between two well-being aims. One has to do with a prerequisite of autonomy: knowledge of a range of possible options. The other is about a kind of disposition formation: induction into fulfilling pursuits. *Theoretically*, a child could be directly inducted in this way into a huge number of activities. But practically, this makes less and less sense the more the number of possible options grows.

In any case, just how many options does the autonomous chooser need to know about if he or she is to flourish? How close do we have to get to comprehensiveness?

I will come back, in the next chapter as well as in Part 2, to the tension between the two aims. Meanwhile, a couple of other issues.

The first goes back to the point that acquiring knowledge of a range of lifestyles should be a *compulsory* requirement. An objector might well use the same sort of argument as I have just relied on. If you want children to be autonomous choosers, this is not something just for their maturity: they need to be apprenticed for this while still young – which speaks for giving them maximum freedom, from the first years of primary school onwards, to choose what they want to do and when.

But why *maximum* freedom? Although some ultras in the world of child-centred education would go for this, it does not seem very sensible. If children are to be *apprenticed* to become autonomous, it follows that they are *not yet* fully there. The younger they are, the less knowledge they are likely to have about possible alternatives. Their apprenticeship will equip them with relevant understanding, gradually give them more experience of making choices of activity, and transform them in other ways too. But no argument, whether based on the rights of the child or anything else, looks likely to justify giving children of 5 upwards *carte blanche* to do what they will without restriction.

The second issue is this. In this section I have been going along with the desire-satisfaction account of well-being and seeing what its curricular implications would be if it were true. But *is* it true? I raised sceptical points about it earlier in the chapter – and in Chapter 8 I pursue them further.

What interests me here is this. Given that secondary-age children – and no doubt even younger ones – are beginning to form ideas about what makes life worth living, how far do they take for granted the very widespread view within the culture that this is entirely up to the individual? How far do they believe that if a person succeeds in getting what they most want out of life, that is all there is to it? Teachers and parents would do well to talk this view through with young people.

I realise the consumer culture in which they and all of us live is not likely to press them towards this kind of reflection. It has a financial interest in getting people to use their free time making choices about goods and serv-ices that satisfy their wants. Its profit margins might be in jeopardy if people began, on any scale, to ask themselves whether want-satisfaction might not, after all, always be the path to a fulfilling life.

All the more reason, then, for educational agencies to undertake this task. I am not saying that they should be trying to engage learners via abstract philosophising. There are plenty of hooks in every student's daily experience that could be used as starting points for discussion or projects.

Chapter 8

Worthwhile activities

1.

Sand-counting has very little, if any, value. Its devotee is certainly successful in getting what he wants, but his desire is incomprehensible. His life is not flourishing but meaningless.

If this is right, one requirement of well-being is that the activities we pursue for their own sakes are worthwhile. But this lands us with another problem – at least as massive as any we have met so far. *What makes* an activity worthwhile?

Let's start small – literally. My wife and I have a little grandson of 17 months – adorable, that goes without saying. Last Sunday his parents brought him to visit us. We spent much of the time playing with him, looking at picture-books, walking with him in the garden to see our little statues, Mr Easter Island and Mr Hercules. If anything was a worthwhile way of spending a day, that was.

How do I know it was? I am tempted to say the question is otiose – no one could seriously ask it. It is like asking the stock philosophical question whether there is really a table in the room. We need to distinguish genuine doubt from philosophical doubt. It may be philosophically helpful to play the sceptic and ask why the table couldn't, after all, be just an illusion; but it is perfectly possible to do this while firmly believing that it exists. It's the same with the family party. It's hard, as I say, to imagine a more fulfilling way of spending one's time. This does not rule out a philosophical enquiry into what makes an activity worthwhile, and I will indeed be coming back to this in Chapter 10. But it does give us a starting-point, something as patently in the middle of the picture as sand-counting is at the edge of it.

It is not too difficult to think of other intrinsically worthwhile activities that can help make up a fulfilling life. Carole goes running in the local fields with her Irish terrier beside her on a lead. Her husband Phil is a gifted carpenter in his spare time: he enjoys making low sitting-room tables out of old railway sleepers. Admittedly, he turns a penny in doing so, but his woodworking is not just a means to an end; it has intrinsic value in itself. A near neighbour of theirs plays guitar in a band and often does gigs across southern England. He and his wife love scuba diving.

I won't multiply examples. One of the striking features about the lives of many ordinary British people today is the wide range of worthwhile activities they enjoy for their own sake. It was not like this 150 years ago, when the country was struggling with the dislocations of the Industrial Revolution. The lives of most people then were miserable. Even for the rich – even for royalty – listening to a concert or seeing a drama were only occasional pleasures. Today, we can all enjoy them at the press of a button on an i-pod or TV.

There is no problem in identifying possible ingredients of a flourishing life. The only difficulty lies in seeing where the task could end. There are so many well-qualified candidates. They cover, as we have seen, relationships as well as activities.

A key consideration in thinking about personal fulfilment is how we spend our time – the minutes, hours and days that make up our life. We are, like other mammals, active creatures. Woven into our activity are longer or shorter periods of passive experience, whether sensations, like feelings of pain, or emotions, like feelings of anger or joy.

It is not enough just to engage in a worthwhile activity for this to count towards one's flourishing. As we saw in Chapter 5, the activity must also be *successful*. Would-be poets deluded about their talents, or endlessly botching carpenters, are hardly thriving. It is the same with relationships. Friendships can go sour. Middle-aged men in love with younger women can be dupes. A personally fulfilling life is one filled with successful engagement in worthwhile activities and with little failure in them.

If you like, this means you have to be a success rather than a failure in life, a winner, not a loser. But this is *not* to say you have to have made a lot of money or held down a job at the top of the tree. This conventional picture has a poor understanding of fulfilment. It is also heartless. It is as if an older way of thinking that divided people into those who will be saved and the rest now has a this-world counterpart. But if we believe that everyone, and not only some, should be helped to make the most of their one life, we need a different starting point. Success is still at the heart of things, but it may well be success in modest, everyday achievements and interactions.

Compare two imaginary lives. The people both earn a living as gardeners, have close relationships with their husbands and children, have many friends, are both keen on bird-watching and cooking. For one of the women all these things turn out well, while the other suffers misfortunes throughout her life, causing her to fall short in most of her relationships and things she does. The first woman has had a more fulfilling life than the second. Her life has been more successful.

This kind of contrast between lives can exist in any human society. We can imagine a traditional tribal society of several thousand years ago, in which two men are both warriors, fathers, brothers, hunters, spear-makers and worshippers of the local gods. As in the previous story, one of them does all these things well, while the other, because of ill health, a series of accidents and other calamities, fails across the board. It is scarcely controversial that the first man has had a more fulfilling life than the second.

Even with some non-human animals, one can make the same kind of distinction. A pet dog who gets on well with family members, is able to romp around the garden and lope around the fields, leads a more flourishing life than one penned up and abused in other ways. Like some other animals, human beings are active, social creatures, whose well-being is a function of how successfully they are able to live as such.

In a modern, liberal-democratic society, successful engagement in worthwhile activities for their own sake is not the whole story. For most of us, these have to be freely engaged in. The warriors in our traditional society had no choice about whether to be warriors, husbands, spear-makers. These were prescribed for them by tribal custom. But in our society we take it as read that it is Carole's choice to go out running with her dog and Phil's to make tables out of sleepers. In our kind of society we enter freely into our sexual and other relationships, choose our own work and non-work pursuits, decide for ourselves our stances towards religion or politics. Personal autonomy is, for nearly all of us, an inalienable component of our well-being.

I say 'for nearly all of us' because not all of us in countries like Britain or the USA value making our life our own. For some religious groups among us, the life we have is not ours but God's. We are on Earth to do what he wills; and well-being, if it exists at all, exists only in another world.

2.

There are three other features of well-being I'd like to mention.

1. Imagine someone, a university lecturer perhaps, who is successful in all the worthwhile projects he undertakes – his teaching, his conference presentations, his chairing of committees. His home life with his wife and children is equally serene and unproblematic. On the account given so far, he is leading a flourishing life, if anyone is. But for some reason he is slightly depressed and this affects everything he does. What he does at work he does well, but it costs him a lot psychologically to force himself to come up to the mark. Even then, there is often something flat and lack-lustre about his performance.

His life is, we will all agree, less than fully flourishing. What is missing, as Joseph Raz (1994: Ch.1) has pointed out in another connection, is wholeheartedness. When his depression lifts, he is able to throw himself into his activities with gusto. He is no longer divided in his attention, thinking partly about the task and partly about himself. He is now able to lose himself in what he does. He is totally absorbed. Everything flows.

It is not only depression that can hold one back. Diffidence, poor self-image or a generally anxious disposition are other possible impediments.

The whole-heartedness requirement embodies the truth in hedonism. Although, for reasons spelt out in Chapter 6, well-being cannot be reduced to pleasurable experience, enthusiastic enjoyment of what one is doing *does* add to one's flourishing. I realise enthusiasm can go too far, as too long spent in the company of the bouncier of one's colleagues can testify. In whole-heartedness, as in many other personal qualities, there is a mean to be struck between extremes.

2. This leads me to the second feature. It is an expansion of the points just made, about personal autonomy and about whole-heartedness. Both of these are virtues – personal qualities – needed for a fulfilled life in a liberal-democratic society. There are others. You must have determination – to carry through something on which you have set your sights; courage – to confront physical and non-physical fears; persistence – to soldier on despite setbacks; and good judgement in making appropriate decisions in particular circumstances, not least when different considerations conflict.

These are only some of the qualities we need in order to thrive. I will be coming back to this in Part 2. As we shall see more fully there, education for well-being is not confined to academic subjects but also develops a range of personal dispositions.

For the moment there is just one more of these virtues that I want to mention. It is needed to counteract the pressures from consumerism and the celebrity culture discussed in previous chapters. We live in a world of temptation. This has come home to us all in recent years in connection with physical desires – for food, drink, sex, sunshine and stimulants. Just as we have to regulate our innate emotions like fear and anger by developing the virtues of courage and self-control, so we have to learn to manage our innate bodily desires. A good upbringing will induct us, for instance, into appropriate ways of eating and drinking – wholesome foods, alcohol in moderation, a freer rein on party occasions, and so on. We learn to protect ourselves from too much sunlight. A frank and sensitive sex education helps us to regulate lust.

Strangely, we do not have a ready word in everyday language to refer to this virtue. The term that philosophers have for it is 'temperance'. The word's associations in ordinary language are most usually with alcohol. Here I shall use it in its broader philosophical sense, to mean the intelligent regulation of one's bodily appetites in general.

Whatever word we use, our present culture needs to highlight the idea behind it. Obesity, anorexia, binge drinking, paedophilia and other forms of sexual abuse, skin cancer and addiction to nicotine, alcohol and other drugs have all become major social and health problems. Many of us, young people especially, are tempted to go too far in all these directions. It is hard to resist urgings from the media, advertising and the internet to indulge ourselves.

We need to acquire the strength of will to resist their temptations. This virtue is closely related to the courage we need to stand out against group pressures to pander to these desires.

It's not only physical temptations. The Methodist church in our high street was totally demolished a few years ago apart from its two spires. These have given its name and its façade to a shopping court. Its outlets are air-conditioned in the summer and warm in winter. You can enjoy cappuccino and almond croissants in the sunshine. Parking is easy. There are loos if you need them, special offers in every shop window and a wonderful bakery for home-made bread and cakes.

The place is irresistible. You go up there because you've run out of tissues and find yourself struggling down the hill with several full carriers... and £65 worse off.

I have used the word 'virtue' frequently in this section. It is an old-fashioned word, not much used nowadays to label the personal qualities I have in mind. This underlines the point made in the Introduction that it is still strange for us inheritors of a moralised, religious culture to feel at home in the new world of well-being. It comes much more naturally to us to use the word 'virtue' as the opposite of 'vice' and synonymous with 'moral goodness' than to use it to refer to desirable personal qualities. As with 'temperance', the challenge is to create a shared vocabulary in which to speak about well-being.

3. My third and final remark is about luck. Good fortune is a *sine qua non* of well-being. A life going well can be blighted by a bad fall, a financial crash, the onset of Parkinson's, imprisonment based on mistaken identity. In the more radical reaches of the Christian world-view from which we are now detaching ourselves, how well you conduct your life has nothing to do with such external circumstances and everything to do with the qualities of moral character displayed in coping with them. The good life, in this picture, is immune to bad luck.

Those of us for whom the mortal life is all there is cannot think like this. That is why we take what steps we can to guard against bad luck or to moderate its consequences. We take out insurance, vote in governments who promise a free health service, safer highways and city streets, controls on the adulteration of food and drink. Some of us, to avoid bad luck, never travel by air, or sit in the sun, use cashpoint machines, or leave the house. But most of us know that a life without ill luck cannot be guaranteed.

Social class also comes into the story. Money and education can cushion misfortune. Reducing inheritance tax means more silver spoons for some babies. Shaping school admission policies so as to favour the better-off reduces the competition their children face in getting into 'good'schools. Better luck for the privileged can mean worse luck for the deprived. If we are interested in a fulfilled life for the many, not the few, this means making life chances more equal across society.

3.

I have been arguing that well-being is not to be understood in terms either of pleasurable feelings or of the successful realisation of our major preferences, however well-informed we are about them. Success comes into the picture, but it is success in engaging in *intrinsically worthwhile relationships and activities*. We all know what some of these are – playing with one's grandchildren, for instance – even though we might find it hard to say in the abstract what makes an activity or a relationship worthwhile. This question is taken up in Chapter 11.

Being successful in this context does not mean being a success in life rather than a failure. The idea is much more ordinary. It applies even to those non-human animals of whom it makes sense to say that they can live life flourishingly. In a liberal-democratic society like our own, it is assumed that most people will want to choose for themselves what activities and relationships they engage in. In this way, personal autonomy enters almost unnoticed into how we conceive of our well-being.

How we get involved in our pursuits is another feature of the latter. Whole- rather than half- heartedness is a *sine qua non*. So are certain personal qualities. To thrive, we need patience, courage, determination, good judgement and a host of other virtues. In a consumerist environment like our own, we need the psychological strength to resist the temptation to buy goods and indulge our physical appetites. To flourish, we also need good luck.

Issues for education

Education has long been plagued by the comprehensive ideal. I'm not referring to a contemporary type of school. What I have in mind goes much farther back – to the seventeenth century, in fact. It took the form then, at least in radical Protestant circles, of giving pupils insight into *every* branch of knowledge, human beings having been made in the image of an omniscient God. These days, we still try to cram the National Curriculum, and the school timetable, with subject upon subject, adding to the traditional collection new demands that children should know about diet, the workings of Parliament, how to use a computer, financial management, religious festivals, entrepreneurship. At classroom level, teachers, often impelled by examination anxieties, try desperately to 'cover the ground'.

We saw in Chapter 7 how a modern kind of encyclopaedism works at a theoretical level to insist that every child *en route* to becoming an autonomous agent should know about the whole range of life choices available. We also saw the downside to this drive for comprehensiveness: that it could well be at the expense of pupils actually engaging in enjoyable activities themselves.

Education for well-being based on the desire-satisfaction view is ill-placed to cater for this engagement. For how will the enjoyable activities be selected? They can't be left, as we have seen, to children's free choices; and if teachers or policy-makers choose them, they risk paternalism. If curriculum activities like science are selected on the grounds that they open a large number of doors to possible life options, what guarantee is there that children will *enjoy* these door-openers rather than put up with them?

This chapter's challenge to the desire-satisfaction view does not make the components of well-being relative to what each individual happens to want. The alternative it proposes is not relative or subjective in that sense. It reminds us that – as we know from our experience of playing with children, listening to music, intimate relationships and craft activities – a fulfilling life is built around successful and whole-hearted, intrinsically motivated involvement in pursuits like these.

Admittedly, this 'like these' points to a longer list of worthwhile activities and kinds of relationships; and questions crop up here about what criteria determine which we include. I come back to these in Chapter 9. The longer the list grows, the more reason there is for making learners aware, as autonomous choosers in the making, of various possibilities open to them. We are thus back with a version of the 'knowing about possible options' educational aim we discussed in the last chapter.

But there is an all-important difference between this version and its predecessor. There is not the same imperative to aim at comprehensiveness. The desire-satisfaction version had to do this because ignoring options that an individual might have chosen looks like paternalism. In the 'worthwhile activities' version, *it matters less* if not every option is known about. Much less weight is placed on comprehensiveness than on engagement.

If we know from the start that a fulfilling life is built around immersion in worthwhile pursuits, we start young people on the road by giving them the experience of fulfilment now. We are less interested in covering syllabuses than in making sure that children are fully, enjoyably and successfully involved in something valuable. This comes first. It is not, of course, everything. We make sure they go on from here to get caught up in other valuable pursuits. Over time they get into all sorts of things – friendships, craft work, exploring nature, reading stories, swimming, gardening, helping other people . . . We give them tasters of activities that we know only some of them are likely to take to in a big way – things like algebra or singing or learning a foreign language. Because we see them as tasters, we do not get upset if they give them up because they can't get drawn into them. That's no problem; there are always other new things to learn that they'll find more fascinating.

We do not expect everyone to leave school with a comprehensive set of competences. We realise they still have perhaps 80 per cent of their lifetime still ahead, and will, with luck, have plenty of time to get into all sorts of other valuable pursuits and relationships. We make sure they get *this* message, too, pointing out to them possible delights ahead, and ways in which they can tap into them through adult education or informally.

It is unrealistic, as I have said, to expect schools and families, taken together, to give children experience of immersion in *every* kind of worthwhile pursuit. But many more can be added to the tally if we bring in the *imagination*. The literary arts, including fiction, drama and film, are ideal media for introducing us to valuable relationships and activities of all sorts that we have not experienced first-hand. So are biographies and memoirs. And when I say 'introducing us', I don't just mean giving us *knowledge* about them in some external way. These artists and writers have the power to make us *feel* what it would be like to live through the loss of a husband and, in time, fall in love again, to climb the world's highest mountains, to hold fast to one's moral integrity through the horrors of a concentration camp. Michael Gove misses out here in his desire to confine the teaching of literature in schools to the 'great tradition' of Dryden and other writers. He overlooks the role that novels and other works, not least those of our own time, can play in vastly expanding our sensitivities to the countless ways in which a fulfilling human life can be lived.

Directly, then, or indirectly via the imagination, families and schools will induct children into all sorts of worthwhile activities and relationships. The pattern will be different from person to person, although we can expect a lot of overlap too. We also expect progression. Success builds on success. Reading simpler stories leads on to reading more demanding ones; getting drawn into a project on life in the Victorian age, to exploring in more detail the rise of the Labour movement or some other historical period.

Success is at the heart of this kind of education. This is not surprising. It is hard to imagine *any* kind of education without some conception of it. Two further examples. One: conventional approaches to education want children to 'do well' at school on the way to 'doing well', financially and vocationally, in the world. Two: an education built around desire-satisfaction as the key to well-being pivots about success in getting what one wants. I'll take these in order.

Wanting one's children to 'do well' in the world is an ancient wish. New England Puritans of the seventeenth century used the same language as middle-class parents today. Cotton Mather's tract, *Cares about the Nurseries*, consists of 'two brief discourses', the second of which offers 'some INSTRUCTIONS for CHILDEN, how they may DO WELL, when they come to Years of Doing for themselves' (Morgan, 1944: 49).

In those days, religious and vocational notions of a successful life were closely intertwined. Indeed, these two categories were inseparable, since to follow one's vocation was to do that which God had called one to do. On one side, then, leading an upright, godly life; on the other, becoming a respected and prosperous farmer, doctor or craftsman. The religious perspective has now largely withered away, but the vocational is more powerful than ever.

As an account of success in life, it needs review, as we saw earlier. Winners imply losers. We need a new vision of society in which everybody can be a success. Melanie Phillips, the British journalist, entitled her book in favour of traditional education *All Must Have Prizes*. But that is not the proper watchword for the alternative urged here. We need a schooling system, and a society, where prizes are less prized – where 'doing well' is available for all, in the shape of successful absorption in worthwhile pursuits.

As for the second example, the notion of success found in desire-satisfaction theory, this has more egalitarian potential than the winners-and-losers version. You don't have to have 'made it' in the conventional sense to have achieved your goals, as long as these are modest enough. But goal-attainment alone is no guarantee of well-being. The life in a Spanish sea-view villa on which one has set one's heart before retirement can prove a disappointment. It may also be short on anything worthwhile.

We need to peel away the false layers around the idea of success, leaving it as success in worthwhile pursuits. In one way, this is not a radical new direction. It is success as most of us know it in our everyday lives. All we have to do is rid ourselves of excrescences around it.

To come back to schools. As things are, they are dominated by a timetable cut up into small pieces. Fifty-minute lessons, sometimes glued together in pairs, become the norm as children get older. There have been understandable, if not now acceptable, reasons for this in the past. A culture that has put a premium on swiftly absorbed, encyclopaedic knowledge has had to find a mechanism for ensuring that every branch of it gets its due.

Confining children's capacity for whole-hearted absorption within bite-sized units is scarcely likely to further it. There is a case for rethinking the timetable and giving this capacity more scope. Some may point to children's limited attention span as a reason for the short-burst timetable. It is, of course, quite true that young children can easily and suddenly give up one thing – playing traffic jams in the sitting-room – for something totally different – kicking a ball around the garden. But this is a world away from the *enforced* change of focus that the standard timetable brings with it. And the 'limited attention span' view fails to accommodate the even more familiar fact, that very often little children have to be *dragged away* from something that thoroughly involves them.

One last thought. Education as induction into worthwhile activities is hardly a brand-new conception. The 1960s saw a celebrated account of this in the work of the philosopher Richard Peters (1966: Ch. 5). But his take on the topic was too narrow. For him, worthwhile pursuits tended to be truth-seeking, like history, science and philosophy. But, important as these are in anyone's education, there are no good reasons for privileging them over all kinds of practical, aesthetic or other activities.

Worthwhile *relationships* as well as activities are constituents of a fulfilling life. Traditionally, schools have seen these as, at most, peripheral, if not obstructive, to their main task. This has been to develop the intellect of each individual learner. That is why school-room furniture often takes the form of rows of separated desks; why tests and examinations are of individual, not collective, achievements; why teachers often prefer their students to engage in the private activity of writing rather than the public one of discussion. Friendships between pupils have been, at best, condoned, not encouraged.

But there is no basis for this. We all know, when not under the spell of theory, that among the most fulfilling experiences of a human life are those of intimacy, friendship and collegiality. Schools have been uncomfortable about promoting them. But why should they be? I take this up again in Chapter 10 and in Part 2. Meanwhile, do factor in – as I suggested a couple of pages ago – the enormous scope schools have to involve children in the world of relationships via the imagination as well as through direct experience.

Chapter 9

Work and well-being

1.

The philosopher G. E. Moore wrote that:

> No one, probably, who has asked himself the question, has ever doubted that personal affection and the appreciation of what is beautiful in Art or Nature, are good in themselves.

> (Moore, 1903: 188)

We do not have to accept his further view that these are the most valuable things in life to agree with him in this.

The houses on the east side of Gordon Square in London now belong to departments of one or other of the colleges of the University of London. Filing-cabinets and anglepoise lamps can be glimpsed through their windows. But the blue plaques on their walls point to the far more gracious existence that went on behind them a century ago. John Maynard Keynes, Lytton Strachey, Virginia Woolf and Clive Bell lived by G. E. Moore's image of the ideal life devoted to friendship and love of beauty.

The Bloomsbury Group were a leisured elite. Few of us can spend as much of our time as they did on their favoured pursuits. But does this mean we cannot lead lives that are equally fulfilling?

A traditional way of thinking about well-being that has come down from Aristotle associates it with the use of leisure. Aristotle himself was writing for a wealthy minority whose basic needs were taken care of by slaves. A later social group, the eighteenth-century British aristocracy, were also a leisure class, pursuing their partying, hunting, garden-making and philandering, with hosts of unseen servants in attendance. Today's pop idols, London-based Russian oil billionaires, and other rich celebrities are their successors.

Even those of us who work for a living often link fulfilment with what we do, or would ideally do, in our free time. There are many of us who wait for the weekend. In this way of looking at things, work is instrumental. Only leisure activities have value for their own sake.

Are we right to think this? Take Phil, the table-maker. His carpentry is a sideline, something he does after work. It is, if you like, a leisure activity. But it is also hard work – as anyone will agree who sees him carrying heavy sleepers on his shoulder down to the big shed he has made at the end of his garden, for sawing, chamfering and drilling.

The neat contrast between leisure and work won't stick. A difficulty is that 'work' gets used in different senses. It refers to the job we do; and also, more broadly, to instrumental activity designed to produce something.

So when we ask what role work plays in human fulfilment, we have to be careful about the sense we have in mind. If leisured people can live flourishing lives, it is not necessary to hold down a job to do so.

This is scarcely news. But what shall we say about work in the other sense, of productive activity? Is *this* necessary to flourishing? Not all forms of worthwhile activity are work. Strolling in the countryside or listening to a string quartet, for instance. In neither case is some end-product intended. Someone might say that one strolls in the woods in order to bring about the end-product of an enjoyable stroll, but this is only a restatement of what the activity is and does not introduce an end-product outside it. You can, of course, be listening to quartets so as to enlarge your musical understanding and sensibility – and, agreed, this does sound like an end-product. But you may also be after purely intrinsic delights, and, if you are, the idea that this is a form of work drops away.

Conversation can be another worthwhile activity enjoyed purely for its own sake. It is interesting that the two kinds of goods that G. E. Moore elevates – personal affection and aesthetic activity – are not necessarily tied to producing something. Could one flourish for a whole lifetime without working in this sense? I don't see why not. Someone could be rich enough to have all her needs met by others and spend all her time in the company of friends, or reading, listening to music, wandering the woods and fields.

Whichever sense of 'work' we take, it is not necessary to human flourishing. But this is not nearly enough to clinch the argument that flourishing depends on leisure, on job-free time.

Leon is a primary school teacher. He especially likes teaching younger children. The work is hard; there is a lot of preparation and marking; and he is not happy with what he sees as an over-emphasis on literacy and numeracy. But he loves his job, enjoys being with little children, encouraging them in their enthusiasms, taking them on trips to the Science Museum and the Sikh temple in Southall, making up songs for them he plays on his guitar... 'It's a wonderful job,' he says. 'I feel I'm being paid for doing something I'd want to do anyway.'

There is an end-product, of course. Leon wants the children to acquire knowledge and skills, learn to work together and extend their sympathies. But his work also brings intrinsic rewards. Many of us, like Leon, get fulfilment from the work we do for a living.

I should make it clear that I'm not talking about just *any* type of buzz that a job can give us. Gogol's meek clerk in his story *The Greatcoat*, Akaky Akakievitch, adores copying documents. He gets huge pleasure from forming individual letters, especially his favourites among them. When he comes to these, his delight is reflected in his face. He chuckles out loud and helps them along with his lips.

Plenty of intrinsic delight here as well as a product to show for it. But is repeatedly copying letters an intrinsically *worthwhile* activity?

Whatever one might say about Akaky, no one would call torturing a prisoner worthwhile. Yet a sergeant responsible for water boarding a terrorist suspect, so that he feels he's about to drown, can adore *his* job, too. Sadists exist.

Let's stick with Leon. At least his paid work is personally fulfilling. It is also, unsurprisingly in our kind of society, self-chosen. I will call it 'autonomous work'.

This should not be confused with autonomy *in work*. Many of us prefer a job with opportunities for self-direction. Although this kind of work is often called 'autonomous', it should be distinguished from autonomous work as I am using the term. A manager in an insurance firm may have plenty of scope in the way she organises her work, but, unlike Leon, may not see it as intrinsically enjoyable. She does it only because it pays well. This is 'heteronomous' rather than autonomous work in my sense.

2.

'Heteronomous' work is work that has *not* been chosen as a major intrinsic goal. It is work that for some reason you have to do. God may have called you to do it. You may have to do it as a slave. You may do it to earn money. As a pupil at school, you may work because your teacher expects this.

Most work is heteronomous. This does not imply that people do not enjoy doing it. Slaves, some factory workers, even some teachers may hate what they do. But others work willingly – the priest carrying out God's work, the business person with a high income and all kinds of fringe benefits, the secretary who likes the company and busyness of the office.

Would it be best if all paid work were autonomous? The trouble is, the real world is not like that. Drains have to be laid, buses driven, carpets hoovered. In any modem society, all sorts of jobs have to be done that few would wish to do unless they had to. Some heteronomous work is unavoidable. But if the social ideal is that every individual should lead a flourishing life, there is a good reason for making whatever heteronomous work there has to be as compatible as possible with this. How?

Heteronomous work, as constrained, is, *prima facie*, in conflict with the ideal of an autonomous life. Insofar as it takes up a large part of one's time – time that could have been used on intrinsically valuable pursuits – it is not good for one's well-being. There is a strong case for reducing it.

How this reduction might come about is a largely practical rather than a philosophical matter, about scope for further automation, for instance. But there are ethical dimensions, too. I am thinking of interconnections between work, the worker's character and the character and well-being of those affected by the work.

Some work is ethically repellent and cannot be undertaken without threat to one's moral integrity. Extorting money from shopkeepers for protection is an extreme example, but any work that treats others merely as means to ends also falls into this category. As well as endangering one's own integrity, it is likely to harm these other people in various ways. The business world of making money, managing, selling, advertising, is always at ethical risk here – which is not to say that codes of good practice and other controls cannot redeem it.

If we turn from the powerful to the powerless, from managers to managed, the case for reducing unpleasant work – work that is mechanical, exhausting, dangerous or boring – in the interests of personal well-being is overwhelming. There is no need to press the familiar point that in a society like ours a lot of work like this goes into producing goods and services – including positional ones – which are superfluous to people's needs and uncoerced preferences, and depend on mass advertising to get us to want them. This wastefulness heaps up behind it an unnecessary mountain of heteronomous work. Individual well-being can be dealt a double blow. The temptations and pressures of consumerism can knock *consumers'* value-hierarchy out of kilter. They can also lead to *producers* spending too much of their lives chained to labouring.

A main reason why heteronomous work militates against personal fulfilment is that it takes up so much of a person's personal time. For most of us alive today, heteronomous work dominates our existence. Broadly speaking, we live to work. This is so both over a lifetime and from day to day. For virtually all of us, each day is nearly completely taken up either with such work or with what is necessary to work effectively – sleep, eating, washing, eliminating, relaxation, recreation.

The centrality of work in our lives has become, over the centuries, a prominent feature of British and American culture, spreading from there across the globe. It has its roots in the Puritan tradition, strong in both countries, with its rejection of the contemplative, or monastic, ideal of the religious life and its revolutionary notion that true Christianity lies in the proper performance of one's daily work. A life of hard, unremitting toil has been seen as a sign of belonging to God's elect. It is a token of salvation. As Tawney (1926) and Weber (1930) have both shown, the Protestant work ethic was closely connected with the early development of capitalism. Religious and economic motives joined forces to weave the new gospel of work into the social fabric.

At a time when this world was less important than the next, the fact that nearly all one's life was spent in unremitting hard work made a certain sense. Now, when most of us believe this life is the only one we have, the hours and days and weeks that compose it are far more precious. They are all we have. If fulfilment is important, it is only in these stretches of personal time that it can take place. This is why we need radically to reconsider the doctrine of work's centrality.

Issues for education

Is school a place for work or a place for learning? We come back to an issue flagged in Chapter 3. The two can come apart: not all work involves learning, and vice versa. This is true in life, and it is true in school.

The most mechanical of jobs – sorting letters, cleaning offices, working in a call centre – may bring no new knowledge with them. Plenty of work here, but, at the limit, no learning. The same can happen in school – from the meaningless rote learning and time-filling exercises in long multiplication now largely in the past, to mind-numbing worksheet activities still with us in the present.

Conversely, in life we acquire all kinds of knowledge and understanding without working at them. You tell me about the three years you have just spent teaching English in Colombia. I happen to tune in to Melvyn Bragg's *In Our Time* radio programme and find out all sorts of things I didn't know about Edmund Burke. Before being physically capable of any productive activity, babies learn all sorts of things about the world through looking at things and hearing sounds around them. Preschool children learn to speak, go on scooters and unlock doors as part of the daily flow of play and social interaction. In schools, pupils find out about human nature and develop in their sympathies and imagination through having stories read to them and getting lost in books they read themselves.

We all know these things, but when it comes to what schools should be doing, we easily forget them. Tradition hems us in. Schools have been places of learning; and they have also been places where children are fitted, practically and intellectually, 'for the work of life'. Those who put the weight on schools as workplaces may not go quite as far as John Wesley, who, as we saw in Chapter 3, said of his new school, 'we do not allow any time for play on any day'. But they still rail on at primary teachers who teach partly through play; and even more so, at those who advocate such methods for secondary schools too.

If we want schools to be sites of valuable learning, we should stick fast to *this* purpose and not let others be entwined around it. The most vigorous of these is the one that has come down to us from Wesley and fellow enthusiasts for the Protestant work ethic. If you think work central to life, you will see schools as seedbeds for this. You will be content with packed timetables, plenty of homework and toiling away for public exams. You will want teachers to work as hard as pupils, setting them an example of how a valuable life should be lived.

The doctrine of work's centrality has coloured educational policy since the nineteenth century and still does so. This is not surprising. Those who shape the policy – politicians, administrators, school leaders – have themselves been inducted into it at school and succeeded later through attachment to it. They are supported by parents who want their children to 'do well', to work hard at school for the sake of a good job afterwards.

Likewise, if, as this book is arguing, the place of work in a flourishing life needs rethinking, the same goes for its place in schools. If valuable learning is to trump diligence, we need to think how this can best occur. Work is bound to figure largely: you can't learn to paint with producing paintings, or to think mathematically without solving problems. If work involves intentional production, it will be a part of schooling at innumerable points: in forming letters of the alphabet, writing essays, conducting experiments, designing a school logo. Some of these things may be examples of the intrinsic worthwhile activities whose centrality to the flourishing life may replace the old centrality of work. Others – like forming one's letters – may equip one with the *wherewithal* to flourish, even if they are not – unless one becomes an Akaky Akakievitch? – constituents of it.

But should work be so salient in school life? How much can children learn through watching films; listening to music; reading for pleasure imaginative literature, biographies, histories; discussing controversial issues; browsing the internet; wandering through the local countryside; engaging in projects that they see as fun? (I am not assuming they do these things without guidance.) I do not know the answer; but if, as seems possible, we are on the edge of a culture shift in which work becomes somewhat more peripheral in our lives, this is worth exploring.

I am reminded in all this of Jacko. Not the superstar, but old Mr Jacottet, who taught me French in the upper reaches of my secondary school. He was good at his job, but even better at getting away from it and letting his humanity and deep-dyed socialism show themselves in talking with us about his memories of the trenches in the Great War, and social injustices nearer to hand. It is a pity that these, the only non-subject-focused discussions I experienced at school, were so much in the margins. I envy those – perhaps still untypical – young people today encouraged to join in structured conversations about sex, politics, the impact of the media, global warming and the meaning of life . . .

I envy, too, those academics and others who, interviewed about their early lives, talk about the hours they spent, when obliged to stay at home for a long period, in reading their way through their parents' extensive collection of books. An early reader myself, I did not come from such a home, but discovered Dickens while at primary school. After age 11, when transferred to my solidly work-centred grammar school, I do not remember reading a single thing more for pleasure. Even today, as a well-schooled workaholic, I need to make a deliberate effort to start reading a novel. It is still work that comes most naturally to me.

It would be good if schools could strike a better balance between work- and non-work-based learning activities. It would be good, too, if they did more to eliminate those grey stretches of time that involve neither work nor learning nor enjoyment.

Film Club points a way forward. In the words of its website, this government-supported initiative 'gives pupils and teachers the chance to explore the world of film through after school film clubs' (http://www.filmclub.org/about-filmclub). With discussion and reviewing among its further activities, it finds a place, but not in the standard curriculum, for perhaps the greatest art form of the last century. The next milestone will be when activities like this are *welcomed into* the school day and no longer left, as poorer relations, outside it.

Work rightly plays a major role in schooling. In line with the discussion earlier in the chapter, priority should go to the autonomous variety. In throwing themselves into productive activities in which they willingly engage and which they enjoy – whether it be solving problems in algebra or the design of furniture or collaborating in a community-based project – students are not only paving a path to their future well-being, they are also experiencing fulfilment now.

Yet so much schoolwork is not of this sort. As something that learners *have* to do, and would not have chosen to do, it is not autonomous, but heteronomous. There is no need to spell out examples. In a system where so much of the curriculum is compulsory, and which the work ethic has pervaded so thoroughly, they are everywhere. We should reduce the amount of non-autonomous work imposed on young people. Living under its dominion strengthens dispositions closer to resentment or resignation than to fulfilment.

Should education be for work or for leisure? If we take 'work' in its widest sense, points made earlier have revealed the false assumption that these are mutually exclusive. What about education for *paid* work, jobs, a career? A book on educational aims in general might have different things to say. But what shall we say in *this* book, which sees schooling through the lens of well-being?

This is a big question. It turns partly on whether we assume the *status quo*, about the amount of time that paid work takes up in one's life, and differences of status between different jobs, or whether we rethink this. I say more about this in Part 2.

For now, I have only two, related, points to make. The first is about life planning. In the English National Curriculum, the new subject Economic well-being and financial capability at Key Stages 3 and 4 (ages 11–16) has 'career' as its foremost 'key concept'. It highlights as a goal 'understanding that everyone has a "career"'. The term is glossed as 'an individual's progression through learning and work'. But is it true that everyone has a career? *Should* everyone have one? Even if most people go for a career, is having one an *essential* part of a fulfilled life? And should young people come to believe that they should use their time at school, and the choices they will be given, partly to plan their future career?

This touches on a wider issue. Some philosophers believe that a flourishing life is one that has to be mapped out – only in broad terms, of course – early on. We all know people who have done this; people, for instance, who decide at 16 that they are going into dentistry, and by 40 will have a leading practice in the West End of London and be celebrated among their peers for their surgical innovations. The question is: is life-planning a non-eliminable part of personal well-being, or is it only an option for those who prefer to arrange things that way?

I spoke in earlier chapters about religious shadows in a secular age. Here we confront another. Life planning is a mandatory requirement according to traditional Protestant attitudes. Your life is not your own, but God's; you have a duty to employ your time on Earth to greatest advantage from a religious point of view. Your duty is to discover the innate talents with which God has endowed you and follow the calling, or vocation, built around these to the utmost of your ability.

But is life planning necessarily a good thing outside a religious framework? We all know people like Becky, who fell in when at secondary school with her parents' urging her to work hard for her exams so that she could go on to a good university and study a sensible subject like medicine or law *en route* to a well-paid job and a comfortable life. In fact, she chose the legal profession, and after her degree at Durham specialised in the lucrative field of employment law. Eight years later, finding no relief from its dullness, she gave it up to become a primary teacher.

Not only can life planning turn sour, it also does not seem to be the *only* way to a fulfilling life. Matt also became a primary teacher in the end and loved the many years he spent in his job. But he never used the maths degree he got at Salford, went off to work in a café in Newquay and hung out with the surfers. After a year or two, he found himself following a girl to Ecuador, teaching a bit of English in Quito and arranging jungle trips for curious Americans. He enjoyed everything he did, in a laid-back, living-for-the-moment kind of way.

If a spontaneous way of life like Matt's can deliver the goods and a planned one like Becky's fails to do so, what should parents and teachers do about life planning? Should they encourage young people in that direction, but with shrewder awareness than Becky had of possible mismatches? Should they try to get them to see the pros and cons of both ways forward – via discussions, perhaps, or via private reading of novels and biographies that bear on this? Should they not get involved at all?

A hundred years ago, most people in a country like Britain wouldn't have been in a position either to life plan or to slip into unstructuredness. Most went into pits, farms, factories and shops as working-class norms dictated. Planning ahead made good sense for aspiring groups above them who had more of a sense of possibilities open to them, while only the very rich or the very bold could afford to take life as it came.

How teachers and parents react to life planning depends to some extent on patterns of employment and quality of life. In Part 2, I say something about rethinking these if our vision for the future revolves around well-being for *everyone*. A society in which the work one does, and school regimes behind this, are less dramatically tied to differences in personal well-being than is the case now, may have less interest in life planning, and more in living for the moment.

Chapter 10

Living the good life: well-being and morality

1.

As we saw in Chapter 2, the 'good life' can mean either the life of moral goodness or the personally flourishing life. In the Puritan tradition, relentless work was straightforwardly a moral duty – no two ways about it. Outside that tradition, work's place in a flourishing life is, as we have seen, far less clear-cut.

Let's now tackle head on the notion of the 'good life'. How does personal fulfilment fit with doing the morally right thing? Is there, indeed, a fit?

Traditional Christianity – and the same is true for some other religions – has always gone for the morally good life. As mortal beings, we should be vigilant followers of God's laws. Personal rewards exist, if at all, in heaven. From this point of view, if we try to promote our own well-being, this can only be a dereliction, a falling away. Instead of living for God, we are living for ourselves.

Non-believers can also put all the weight on moral goodness – those, for instance, who flex every sinew in the cause of social justice or the rights of animals and see all other ways of spending their time as selfish.

In both its religious and secular versions, the view seems to rest on the assumption that we act either for moral reasons or out of self-interest. There are only these two sources of motivation. Is the assumption sound?

Admissions to hospital accident departments plummeted on the weekend when the last Harry Potter book was published. Rather than going out on their bikes and scooters, children stayed in their rooms super-glued to its pages. What was their motivation? Few, if any, had furthering their own well-being in mind. Few, if any, were reading the book out of moral concern. I suspect that 99 per cent of them just wanted to get into the story, to see how events unfolded. Their reasons were intrinsic to the activity, not extrinsic to it.

It is not true, then, that reasons for action must be either for moral ends or to do with furthering our own interests. The picture is more complex. There are reasons falling outside both categories.

Take another kind of case. Think of someone who believes that eating sweets is bad for him but is always being tempted to buy them. He's patently not doing this for moral reasons, but neither is he doing it for self-interested ones. He is simply succumbing to a strong desire, with no further goals in view. In this way you could say that he is like the Harry Potter readers. Having read earlier Harry Potter books, they just want to get hold of the latest one. They, too, are powerfully motivated by a present desire, without any thought of how this might increase their overall well-being.

If this is right, and there are not just two kinds of motivation, promoting young people's well-being does *not* imply encouraging them to look out for Number One. For suppose something like the account of well-being in Chapter 8 is correct: a flourishing life is one in which you successfully and whole-heartedly engage in worthwhile activities and relationships. For it to be flourishing, *you don't have to aim at your flourishing*; you can be motivated by features of the activities and relationships themselves. Just as the Harry Potter readers wanted to see what happens in the story, so others of us may want to spend time with an old friend from Chile, or watch what happens to the sweet pea seeds we have planted, or spark an interest in nonsense verse in the primary school children we are teaching. All these things can make our lives more fulfilling. In no case need we be doing them with a self-interested goal in mind.

If this is right, there is no quick route to the strenuous conclusion that whatever we do we should do for moral ends, not self-interested ones. These two kinds of motivation do not exhaust the field.

2.

This line of argument also casts doubt on whether we should be opposing moral goodness and personal fulfilment in the first place. Go back to the teacher in the primary class. Her work is personally fulfilling. A main reason for this is that she is engaged in the morally laudable activity of helping children to learn things. In this example, being moral is not at odds with one's own thriving: it is one of the forms that one's own thriving can take.

Is this too quick? There is a view of morality that says that the kind of loving concern motivating the schoolteacher lacks what it takes for her actions to be morally right. For this she needs a different kind of intention. She needs to act out of a sense of duty. She needs to behave towards her pupils as she does because this is the morally right thing to do.

But I can't see any good reason for favouring the duty-bound view. If I were a married woman, I would rather my husband was kind towards me because he was fond of me rather than because he believed he had a moral obligation to behave in this way. Children, too, are likely to respond better to a teacher who, at an emotional level, really cares for them than someone driven by a sense of duty.

From now on I shall understand morality in the less restricted sense. It has to do with protecting or promoting others' well-being. Another word for it is altruism. Agreed, this rules out the view, more prominent in the religion-steeped world of my youth than now, that it is morally wrong to masturbate, but that may be no great loss.

A link between morality and well-being is also apparent in the area of basic moral rules. Take the idea that it is morally wrong to lie. In the Judaeo-Christian framework, this goes back to one of the ten commandments and our duty to obey it. In a non-religious setting, we can still believe in the immorality of lying, but see the reason for it in the fact that lying tends to get in the way of others getting on with their lives as they wish. It makes it more difficult for them to thrive. On this view, the point of familiar moral injunctions about telling the truth, keeping promises, refraining from injury etc. is to make it easier for others to lead a fulfilling life.

On this understanding of morality, then, we have no good reason to think that it is necessarily at odds with personal well-being. The caring primary school teacher shows that it need not be.

Are we yet out of the wood? Aren't clashes between morality and self-interest still possible? Can't there be cases where if I do what is good for me I may be going against the interests of other people, and vice versa?

Gauguin famously left his family to paint in the South Seas. Shall we say that it was *morally wrong* for him to leave them, but at the same time *good for him* to do so? Is there not the starkest of all conflicts here between the two?

But do we have to characterise the conflict in this way? It is not – I shall presume – as if Gauguin was not fond of his wife and children and that he had only stayed with them out of a teeth-gritting attachment to duty. Perhaps he loved them very much and their life together was part of what made his own life so fulfilling. His dilemma may well have been that art had a stronger hold on him.

Describing things this way makes the conflict *internal* to his well-being. It is not a conflict between his well-being and morality. He had to choose between two worthwhile pursuits since they could no longer be carried on together. Apart from the fact that it is a much more dramatic example, this is in the same league as, say, the person who, because she is short of time, gives up her gym membership to leave more time for her allotment. Ordinary life is full of conflicts like this.

Can there be clashes between morality and one's own well-being that *cannot* be re-described in this way? Suppose you are about to leave home to be interviewed for a marvellous job as a blues singer for which you are the front runner. An elderly couple, who are strangers to you, are passing by your house. The husband drops dead of a heart attack and you spend the rest of that day comforting his widow and seeing to arrangements. As a result, you miss getting the job, which has to be given to someone else.

Is *this* a case that can only be depicted as a clash between moral demands and one's own interests? I don't think so. If your well-being is a function of successful engagement in worthwhile activities, the good work you did on the widow's behalf *could* count towards this.

But what about this? In a small town somewhere in the middle of the USA, a resentful ex-pupil of the local high school bursts into a class and is about to gun down the woman teacher against whom he has a grudge. A student rushes to protect her and is killed by the bullet meant for her teacher. Altruism can hardly coexist with what is good for the heroine in this case – at least from a post-religious perspective. The victim is, after all, no longer with us.

There may indeed be limiting cases like this where altruism and well-being have to come apart. But for the most part, they need not. For all of us, relationships play a part, usually a big part, in our welfare. Doing things for friends, family members, neighbours, colleagues, even strangers need not be at a cost to ourselves, even when it means interrupting or abandoning some project we have on the go. Sure, this involves switching to another kind of worthwhile activity, but then we often move on to other projects even when there is no urgent demand to help someone else.

3.

Apart from relationships, many of our activities involve some kind of co-operation with others for shared goods. This again challenges the conflict in question, that between altruism and one's own good. A flute-player in an orchestra wants the concert to go well. Its doing so is good for her and good for her colleagues, to say nothing of the audience. It is not as though the benefits to each individual can be separately attributed, so that altruistic benefits to other players can be separated out from those accruing to the flute-player alone. If the whole concert is a success, the sharing of well-being is indivisible.

So many day-to-day activities fit this pattern – working in a team to make a bathroom, to care for patients, produce a newspaper, cultivate vegetables, teach children. Even where the newspaper goes bust or the cauliflowers all wither, there are still the varied benefits of working together – the giving and receiving of mutual recognition, losing oneself in a common task, shared enthusiasms and consolings.

Closely related are the personal qualities, or virtues, we prize in those with whom we share an activity. We value being with people who are, for instance, independently minded, resilient, good-humoured, ready to see the other's point of view, or to go the extra mile.

Speaking of virtues, it has always seemed to me odd to classify them, as some philosophers have done, into 'self-regarding' ones like temperance and 'moral' ones like honesty or generosity. Given the salience of social activity in all our lives, it is good *for me* to be an honest or generous friend or colleague, just as it is good for you in many ways if I keep my physical desires under appropriate control.

I have been talking about co-operative activities like teaching and farming. How far does this category stretch?

Think for a moment of more solitary pursuits that may add to a person's fulfilment – writing poems, looking at pictures, listening to music, wandering through an attractive city, cycling, birdwatching, philosophising, growing dahlias. It is true that all these things can be done on one's own, unlike playing in a football match or working as a nurse. But they cannot be understood as atomic activities in which other people are not involved. Writing a novel is engaging in a specific form of art-making, a form with a tradition, a history, its own conventions and criteria of excellence. Becoming a novelist is entering into an apprenticeship, becoming a participant in a social practice. There are others around you, just as there are others around you if you become an engineer or a lawyer. They are not physically with you on a daily basis. The novelist works alone in her cottage, it is true, but she works among a legion of unseen fellow participants – other novelists working today, novel readers, teachers and learners of literature, publishers and critics, as well as writers, readers, publishers and critics from the past and still to come.

The well-being of the solitary novelist is promoted insofar as she is successfully and whole-heartedly engaged in her worthwhile pursuit. What is this pursuit? What is she trying to achieve?

It is impossible to characterise this without bringing in some kind of shared interests. Even where her main aim is to explore her own inner life, the streaming of her consciousness, she is doing this in such a way that others can profitably read her. She is shaping, organising her material with their interests and expectations partly in mind. She is working, too, within a certain tradition of novel writing, which has Proust, Joyce and Virginia Woolf among its architects. Given that she is a serious writer, she cannot but relate her own work to this heritage. She is aiming to write a good work within this genre, one which will help it to bear fruit, perhaps in a new form. Her task, too, is a shared one.

Although I have been urging the impossibility of putting one's own well-being in one compartment and that of others in another, I wouldn't want anyone to infer from this that being a painter or a birdwatcher is all that one has to do to lead an altruistically sensitive life. For this, there are other values that should weigh with all of us, including what are often called moral values like truthfulness, respect for others and justice. I am reluctant to call them 'moral' – rather than 'prudential' or 'self-interested' – because, as a citizen who pursues with others the shared ends involved in creating a decent society, being trustworthy, considerate and fair is as much a feature of my own well-being as it is of yours.

4.

I have tried to challenge the traditional view that morality and self-interest are necessarily in conflict with each other. In a post-religious age we need to reconceptualise their relationship. When we do so, we see that at the heart of morality is concern for others' well-being rather than dutiful obedience to laws thought to be of divine origin. Once this shift takes place, it becomes easier to see that in many, perhaps most, of our activities that bring us personal benefit, this benefit is closely interwoven with that enjoyed by other people. In addition, situations where responding to moral demands on us seems to be at the cost of our own flourishing, can often, if not always, be re-described so as to avoid this consequence.

The discussion has also revealed a flaw in the traditional argument that morality, as traditionally understood, has to be one's only lodestone, seeing that the only other possible motivation is the pursuit of self-interest. The flaw in this is that one can also be motivated by features intrinsic to an activity. The significance for a post-religious culture is this: *for people to lead a flourishing life, they do not have to have this as their goal.* They can find themselves *caught up* in valuable relationships and activities and thrive as a result. This does not rule out having as one of their aims leading a flourishing life, but if they do so, the question arises what benefit this motivation brings one over and above the intrinsic forms of motivation described.

A final point is this. If morality has to do with concern for others' well-being, what does this concern consist in? It is partly about helping them to satisfy their basic needs. It is partly about protecting them from further harms like being deceived, injured or robbed, and about sympathetic identification with them in various forms of distress. And it is partly about enabling them, where appropriate, to take part in worthwhile activities, including relationships. In this third concern, we have to be careful to avoid paternalism. We should not be steering others into some specific activity we feel would be good for them. And we should not be getting them to believe that they would be falling short if they did not pursue their own well-being. As we have seen, one does not have to have this motive in order to thrive. But quite apart from this, people should be left free to make what they will of their lives, even if they knowingly spend it on what is worthless.

Issues for education

If schools made pupils' well-being central, this might upset those for whom the cult of self-concern has already gone too far. But this way of looking at things contains several misconceptions.

Suppose some teachers do indeed encourage the pursuit of self-interest. Perhaps they remind pupils that it is a harsh, competitive world out there.

Perhaps they urge them to make option choices for their GCSE and A-level courses that boost their chances of landing a well-paid job.

Are they necessarily furthering their well-being? They may be reinforcing the dubious idea that this can only be a competitive good. They may be steering them towards curriculum subjects they come to hate, having chosen them not out of love but for future gain. They may be getting them to believe, falsely, that in order to lead a flourishing life they have to *aim* at leading one.

The first misconception is that if a school promotes pupils' well-being, it must be encouraging them to look out for their own interests.

This is not true. If it gets a child thoroughly absorbed in some worthwhile pursuit – listening to jazz, say – this is likely to be personally beneficial to them. Yet this has nothing to do with appealing to self-interest, since the motivation is *intrinsic* to the activity.

A second misconception is not far behind. This is the false assumption that personal well-being and moral goodness are somehow opposed to each other, that an emphasis on one must be at the expense of the other. What is there opposed to moral goodness in getting caught up in the world of jazz?

'Moral goodness' can mean different things to different people. Some link it to living an upright life according to moral principles, perhaps religiously based, perhaps not. Others have a less law-like conception and see it more in terms of acting on the feelings of warmth and sympathy one has for other people. Whichever view one takes, it is hard to see how getting involved in music or in any other worthwhile activity must make one any less of a moral being.

It might even *strengthen* one's moral dispositions. If we understand these in the second sense, in terms of altruistic feelings and behaviour, then, as we saw earlier, many of the worthwhile activities into which schools can induct children are co-operative pursuits in which *my* well-being and *your* well-being are indivisible. Playing in an orchestra, working together on a science experiment, or in a project on medicine in the local community, furthers each child's well-being *through* the bonding that takes place with others.

I don't know if a person could lead a personally fulfilling life if they had *no* concern for other people. Some think this possible. Imagine, for instance, a psychopath totally locked up in his own world of advanced mathematics, which he pursues with zest while being utterly manipulative towards all his acquaintances. But whatever one says about this issue in the abstract, as teachers and educationists we have good reason to come down on one side rather than the other. It may or may not be logically possible for the concept of personal well-being to exclude altruism, but it makes good sense for schools to keep the notion of well-being that *they* use inextricably intertwined with it. This is because they rightly have an interest in the moral education of their pupils and want them to act altruistically. In principle, they could hive off this side of their work under a separate category from their work in advancing each child's well-being; but for reasons I have already mentioned, this would be extraordinarily difficult to do. I cannot, in any case, think of any plausible reason why they might want to do it.

Activities that help others to enjoy good health, or life above the poverty line, or freedom from oppression, or an interesting life, are worthwhile pursuits if anything is. As such, following the argument of Chapter 8, it benefits *the agent* to engage in them, provided he or she does so with commitment and successfully. This is true of an older school student who chooses options in science with a view to becoming a medic; or of a pupil lit up by the citizenship work she is doing on overseas aid.

Citizenship is one of the three National Curriculum subjects that bear directly on moral education. The others are *Religious education*, and *Personal wellbeing*. All three directly and explicitly cover, among other things, the development, reinforcement, or discussion of moral/altruistic attitudes. These also feature in other subjects, if less prominently, as well as in pedagogy and school ethos.

What picture of morality and its relation to their own well-being are students likely to pick up from these different sources? This is an empirical question to which I do not have an answer. But I'm willing to wager that the picture will not always be a clear one.

In the last half of the twentieth century, schoolchildren must have often been confused about what it meant to be a morally good person and how they could become one. Was it their duty to do as much as they could for other people, or was it enough for them to get on with their own affairs as long as they refrained from lying, cheating, physically or mentally abusing others or otherwise interfering in their lives? Should their morality, in other words, be maximal or minimal?

This was a time when organised Christianity was fast on the wane in Britain. Children were brought up to believe it is wrong to kill, injure, lie, break promises or be unkind or unchaste. They knew they should forgive wrongdoers and help others in distress. But the old backing for these rules was on the way out. Those of us brought up around the middle of the century and later still felt a strong sense of obligation to do or refrain from these things. We still felt the same age-old guilt when we did wrong. But what was the system into which all this fitted? What, for the godless, were its foundations?

Now, some way into the twenty-first century, the old shadows are still with us. Some schoolchildren still get their morality, well packaged, from their religion. The less- or non-religious still grow up in faith's moral heritage. But the culture is changing. In 1950 there was no sign of a major challenge to how one thought about morality. Now, in 2010, a powerful alternative is already at work. It sees our ethical life with others not so much in terms of duties, rules and principles, but more built around dispositions, inculcated from childhood, like kindness, friendliness, helpfulness, trust, tolerance and fairness.

This alternative perspective draws no sharp line between personal well-being and altruism, recognising that so many of the activities that are intrinsically beneficial to us personally – like being a teacher – also benefit others, very often intentionally so.

Schools need to tidy up what they provide on the ethical front. The present lack of co-ordination is not helpful. In all but the most clear-sighted schools, pupils are likely to have less than well-thought-through ideas about how they should behave towards others and how this might relate to their own well-being. Schools should not be in the business of sowing confusion. On the contrary, their business is with bringing light to dark places. If they employ three, four or more vehicles of ethical teaching – RE, *Personal wellbeing*, *Citizenship*, school ethos, ethical aspects of literature, history and other subjects – they have a responsibility to see that all these curricular vehicles work together in the interest of clarity and enlightenment.

Chapter 11

Are there experts on well-being?

1.

A personally fulfilling life is one replete with successful engagement in worth-while activities. These, I argued in Chapter 8, are not relative to individual preferences. But what grounds can be given for this non-relativity? Is well-being *objectively* determinable? And if so, how?

Perhaps via biology? Flourishing is different for different species. Cats do well if there are trees around up which to scamper; elephants don't go in for climbing. Human beings share some sources of well-being with other creatures, but, being differently constituted, not others. It is not difficult to link standard candidates for worthwhile activities with features of our nature. We enjoy physical exercise. If we were made of different stuff, this might have no attraction for us. We are social and sexual animals and also self-aware ones. So the high value we attach to intimate relationships is hardly surprising. Cats can see and hear things, but they lack the self-aware-ness in doing this that human beings possess. They cannot *dwell* on what they see and hear, separate off some sights and sounds as particularly delec-table. We human beings can. It is the foundation of our attachment to the arts and natural beauty. Sea eagles on the island of Mull look after their young in their treetop nests, bringing them whole carcasses of sheep and tearing off morsels for them until they learn how to do this for themselves. We, driven less by instinct and more by foresight, find fulfilment in using our rational powers to bring up our children, as well as in teaching and childcare. Some other animals are curious by nature, but it is the higher-order, self-awareness-dependent form of curiosity that human beings have that opens the door, for us but not for them, to history, mathematics, psychology and all other branches of knowledge.

There must be *something* to the notion that human well-being depends on human nature. We saw this, too, in the sphere of basic needs. If we were not constituted in the way we are, if we were tin people, we would not have to have oxygen, homes, clothes, food and drink.

The issue is whether we can read off what it is to flourish from facts about what sorts of creatures we are. For instance, can we base friendship and love of music on our human nature? It is hard to see how. True, we are social animals and we have the power of hearing; but social animals can be capable of sadism as well as friendship. Having ears, we can pick out raucous and painful sounds as well as musical ones. Disvalues as well as values depend on our natural abilities.

We need a more solid basis for why an activity is worthwhile. Looking at aesthetic values may help. They include the sheer sensuous beauty of sounds and sights, as well as formal qualities to do with balance, contrast and complexity; and qualities more directly connected with human concerns, such as expressiveness, humour and depth of insight into human nature.

What is the basis for these values? They are not simply a function of personal preference. Although different individuals may weight them differently, they exist independently of private inclinations. Neither, drawing on reasons just given, is their attractiveness derivable from our human nature.

They are qualities discovered in works of art and other aesthetic objects by competent judges in the field. The qualities exist independently of any particular person's inclinations. Not everyone may at first perceive them. We need practice in doing so. Experienced judges can induct us, bring us, for instance, to see the way an unexpected longer line in a poem about a skylark mirrors the expansiveness of its melody.

Aesthetic values in their present abundance are largely the product of the last few centuries. Not that this period has been static. New values have been added to a growing canon. Specifications of more general values have arisen. Values have coalesced and overlapped with others to form qualities appreciated independently. Many of these changes have occurred through the introduction and development of new art forms.

The novel is one of these, being largely the product of the last three centuries or so. The question, What are the features of a good novel? simply could not have been asked before then. As the form has developed and generated sub-species, more specific values have come into existence – those to do, for instance, with a good detective novel. Music has proliferated into a multitude of forms and genres, both classical and popular. Gardens and landscapes have become the focus of aesthetic interest in their own right. Film is now a new art form with its own canons of excellence, overlapping with those of drama, other visual arts and an aesthetic interest in nature.

There is no need to generate more examples. The main point should be clear. Aesthetic values are extra-individual. They cannot be understood except as historically located, the product of a culture. This is not to say that, once in existence, they cannot persist outside the cultural conditions that produced them. They can outlive these. The new qualities that Mozart added to classical music did not die with the princely regimes of the eighteenth century. The fact that they are cultural in origin does not mean that aesthetic values are relative to certain cultural conditions.

Aesthetic activities suggest a way forward for worthwhile activities more generally. Being a clinical psychologist is a form of work unknown much before the twentieth century; working on a computer help desk was unknown much before the twenty-first. Both can be fulfilling; both bring with them their own specific values. Helping others, possessing and intelligently applying knowledge, and so on, are not, in their general form, unique to them, but the particular form they take and the way they are combined *are* unique.

The last two centuries have seen a vast proliferation in fulfilling kinds of work, most of them unknown in a pre-industrial age. (They have also seen a huge expansion of *un*fulfilling forms of labour.) Extend the period back a century or two and you find equally impressive changes in intimate relationships. The modern idea of marriage as something freely entered into by both parties and based on love and companionship is an institution with roots partly in sixteenth- and seventeenth-century Puritanism. This pattern of married love, in its turn, has generated further variants: companionate marriages, open marriages, stable unmarried partnerships, gay and lesbian unions.

Field after field tells a similar story. Think of inventions and variations in sports and outdoor activities over that period. Think of developments in home-making, in gardening, in foreign travel, in scholarship, in teaching, in socialising, in bringing up children.

It is not surprising that I keep coming back to changes within the last 400 years or so. It is over this period that the idea that life is not a passage to another state, but has its own intrinsic significance, has gradually gained ground.

Personal flourishing is not, as market theorists and others would have us believe, a matter of an individual's desire-satisfaction. Its ingredients are not relative to our particular wishes; they lie outside us as individuals, are created largely within cultures.

Are there some values that escape the cultural net – values more directly dependent on the way we are made? We enjoy listening to birdsong, smelling the scents of flowers, sexual activity, wandering about in the sunshine. Pleistocene Man could have enjoyed all these things too – even if he could not have enjoyed watching surf movies or clubbing.

I don't want to deny this, not knowing much about life in the Pleistocene, although I suspect it was less laid back than these examples suggest. In our own case, these enjoyments are often more convention-bound than they may seem. The flowers in whose scents we delight are carefully placed to produce just this reaction, in herbaceous borders and in living-room vases.

As with aesthetic values, life values, more generally, are not relative to the culture in which they were formed. We may owe the institution of marriage based on affection partly to the Puritans, but it is still important to us, even though its religious connotations are now largely forgotten.

2.

If individuals are not authorities on what a flourishing life is for themselves, who – if anyone – is? Cultures may generate worthwhile activities. But they also spawn activities with little value, like playing the lottery, as well as activities with significant disvalue – slavery, children working down mines, pushing drugs. Cultures also land us with misleading conceptions of well-being – the hedonist and desire-satisfaction theories already discussed. It is because of culture that so many of us are confused about the good life. Who will sort us out? Where are there ethical experts?

There are plenty of takers. Lifestyle and personal counsellors: Sunday supplement journalists, purveyors and promoters of health regimes, yoga teachers, best-selling writers on meditation, saffron-robed converts, new age, new faith gurus, bishops bigging up our confusions so as to shepherd us back to Jesus.

Philosophers? This gets a bit near the bone. Are we to be lumped in with the sham salvationists? The approved, pious answer from our trade is that we are different. We don't claim some superior vision. We can't tell you to go for this way of life rather than that. We don't advocate a regime of joss-sticks and soya milk. We disentangle the general concept of well-being, not the knots in any individual's pursuit of happiness.

I think this is basically right. Pied pipers may exist in our ranks, but they are few. Our interest is in conceptual structures and in sound or unsound patterns of argument. Getting one's thought in neater order is what some people find they need – and philosophy can really help here. I know from my own experience as a young man how liberating an exposure to hard, academic philosophy can be. The swirls of confusion inside my head were stilled. Ideas that tramped around my inner universe, attaching themselves to this then that, never knowing where their home might be, formed up, touched fingertips, arranged themselves in straight lines.

On late summer evenings, bees, wasps, flies, moths, dragonflies – and once a magnificent peacock butterfly – fly into the cellar where I work and can't find their way out again into the garden. I turn off the strip lighting, open the door wide, turn on the patio light outside and coax them into liberty. Philosophy can do this too. It can show you the way out of muddles – and in so doing set you free. What it does not, or should not, do is tell you specifically in which direction then to fly. It is in this that it differs from other guides.

Who, then, is an expert on how well any individual is thriving? To whom can we turn? No one can lay down in detail how a person should best live. There are simply so many ways of thriving, so many forms of well-being goods.

But are there authorities, more generally, on the ingredients of personal flourishing? The arts, again, may throw light on this. Despite disagreements among critics, objectivity *is* at work in their field. Their judgements are justified by arguments, always open to replacement by better ones.

I realise this is an ideal picture and that actual critical judgements do not always follow this sober pattern. But there are plenty of critics dedicated to producing well-founded accounts of the strengths and weaknesses of works in their field. They see themselves as belonging to a serious community of enquirers.

Their communities each have histories. Over the past 200–300 years, expertise has been built up in literary criticism, music criticism and other fields. Here is a stock of opinions that can help people today to form their own judgements.

In making these judgements, some people are thus better placed than others. Someone who has never read Russian poetry is in a worse position to judge the value of Pushkin's *Bronze Horseman* than someone who has studied the subject for years and is an accepted authority. I, who have an amateur interest in the field, cannot vie with the latter but can make a better fist of things than the former.

This gives us a template: outsiders, more authoritative insiders, ordinary insiders. Can we apply it, more generally, to judgements about the components of well-being? Here there are next-to-no complete outsiders. Nearly everyone gains some experience of friendship, for instance. But all of us are outsiders *vis-à-vis* some pursuits, indeed most pursuits. I know nothing of Persian music; you are ignorant of chemical engineering. In insidership and outsidership we find all sorts of gradations. An important factor here is social class. My father-in-law, who spent most of his days with his head inside the bonnet of motor cars he was repairing, discovered the world of the visual arts in his seventies, got a good pass in A-level Art and became fascinated by the work of artists like Turner. There have been and are many working-class people in Britain for whom most literature, serious music, visual art, science and history, as well as whole ranges of rewarding professional jobs, are closed books. There may be very few complete outsiders; but there are many – monstrously too many – people whose horizons are very limited.

Turning to more authoritative insiders, is there any parallel in the sphere of well-being to critics in the arts? John Stuart Mill held, as we saw in Chapter 3, that the mental pleasures of intellectual and aesthetic activity are of higher value than physical pleasures, because those who know both kinds of enjoyment markedly prefer the former. The argument is unconvincing for several reasons, not least the absence of empirical evidence in its support. If it had been sound, we would have made progress in identifying authoritative judgements on the flourishing of particular lives. We would have known that a life rich in mental pleasures is higher in well-being than one less favoured.

There does not seem to be a case for a relatively easily demarcatable group of well-being critics, unlike the situation in the arts. There is no community of experts on what constitutes a flourishing life. Sure, there are plenty of gurus around, as I have said. But there is no good reason to believe them.

What *is* true in Mill is that some people are in a better position than others to know about well-being goods. Those who know nothing about jazz, or skiing, or close friendship, or working as a vet are obviously in a worse position than those inside these activities. The most authoritative voices on what constitutes our well-being are among those with a wide acquaintance with all sorts of goods.

The closest we can get to authorities is a far looser body of people than a well-demarcated community of experts. They must not only have some experience of most major areas of worthwhile activity, but also be interested in reflecting on what makes a flourishing human life, on which candidates are genuine ingredients and which will-o'-the-wisps. They must be people who have some knowledge about all these things and also some freedom of spirit in which to do their thinking. Some do this in a more solitary way than others, but, like art critics, all welcome critical discussion of their ideas.

Two centuries and more ago, those who fitted this bill were largely confined to the rich and those associated with them, and not by any means to all of these. We are talking about the more reflective among them, about people with wider interests than country pursuits, or making money, or following the conventions of their circle.

Nearly everyone must have been outside this group. The situation is very different today in Britain and comparable countries. Few of us have our horizons hemmed in by extreme poverty, drudgery or constricting conventions. Few are so occupied in meeting our basic needs that we have no time for anything else. Most of us, including many of the least educated, have been exposed to a huge array of well-being goods, some experienced directly, others via the imagination. They include the affections of family life, friendship, sexual relationships and other forms of companionship; occupational goods; sport and exercise; home care and garden care; an interest in other animals; travel at home and abroad.

The arts deserve a comment to themselves. Television has brought comedy, drama, soap operas, dancing and pop concerts into all our homes. Music of every genre is easily accessible, wherever and whenever we want it. What was, even in royal circles in the early twentieth century an occasional treat – a visit to the theatre or to listen to music – is now a daily possibility for a whole population.

All these and other kinds of worthwhile activity are within reach of most of us. And this is only a minimum. Thanks to educational improvements, many of us engage in further artistic, intellectual and other pleasures, to which others, like my father-in-law before his retirement, have had no access.

There are no sharp edges here, no higher and lower culture, only complex spectra of involvement across whole populations. We also enjoy thinking and talking about what we like and don't like about our activities, comparisons between them, conflicts we face in doing one thing rather than another. So on the back of first-order valuable activities comes the higher-order – but not necessarily higher-value – activity of reflecting about these, alone or with others.

The latter is not always face-to-face, as in conversations we have with friends and colleagues. We also listen to what novelists, dramatists, poets, biographers, academics, press and TV commentators have to say. At their best, they help us to clarify or concretise our own more inchoate thoughts about well-being, challenge them and add new perspectives. As creators of public texts and events, they provide us with shared reference points and illustrations. You might even say they help to keep going a national, and sometimes international, conversation, which all of us can drop into and out of as we wish.

Three hundred years ago, opinion-formers were few. Today there are so many more participants in worthwhile activities and in reflection on them; so many more commentators; so many more worthwhile activities themselves.

Where, then, can we find authoritative voices on the content of well-being? As with political authority in our age, they do not belong to an aristocracy or to any other social group. They are diffused across the population. In democratic politics, we each have, in theory, an equal voice in determining what kind of society we want. Our participation as electors is formalised, brought under clear rules. Involvement beyond this role varies from person to person. It is more difficult to pin down. If I am right that nearly all of us can now add to the discussion about flourishing, this is also in an unformalised way. There are no rules laying down that we should all have an equal say. Yet there are no well-being experts whose voices legitimately crowd out others. Nearly all our voices are heard, in different contexts and to differing extents.

Well-being is not to be understood in terms of individual desire-satisfaction, even where the desires are both informed and of major significance in a person's life. It is not subjective in this sense. But neither is it an objective matter, to do with derivation from features of our human nature. The truth is more subtle. Well-being is still desire-dependent, but the desires in question are those not of an individual but of the looser collection of people described in the last paragraph.

It is hard to be precise about who is inside this body, and if inside, how far inside. I have been emphasising that nearly all of us are inside to some extent, that those who have a fuller acquaintance with different kinds of goods are further inside than others, but that there are no sharp lines at any point.

This is where education comes in. One of the purposes of education in a democratic society is to equip people for a flourishing life. As part of this aim, they also become better qualified to make judgements about human flourishing. They become better-informed contributors to the national and global conversation.

All this is part of education for democratic citizenship. The link is not hard to see. A citizen is expected to participate, as an elector and in other ways, in decisions about the future of a political community. These decisions are about how to make life better for people, about their flourishing. The more fully the citizen understands what this involves, and the less he or she is led astray by misconceptions of it, the better for the polity.

I will come back to educational matters in a moment. Meanwhile, I hope the main theme of this part of the argument has come through clearly enough. In the European context at least, well-being goods have been increasing in range and specification for several centuries. As they have grown, those people who are best placed to know about them have also changed.

Someone living in 1850 may, if fortunate, have been well fitted to understand what it was to live a thriving life in the mid-nineteenth century. But he or she could hardly be a reliable judge – at least in any detail – of what this would be a century and a half later. Those of us living today are obviously in a better position. Not all, but many of us. The last century and a half has seen a broadening of participation here, parallel to developments in political democracy. There is still some way to go on both fronts. Dykes continue to be erected by those who see themselves at the top end of society to keep those 'below' from sharing in the good life and in political power. Whether the dykes will continue to be breached over the next century is uncertain.

Issues for education

How far should schools and families help pupils think about the *backing* for ideas about well-being? It is true that they have a more pressing task: to get children fully absorbed in the components of well-being themselves. Induction into worthwhile activities and relationships must be the first priority. To take a parallel case, a parent brings up her very young children to be considerate by encouraging considerate behaviour. At the outset, they are not expected to understand *why* this is important, but she begins very early to drum it home that other people count too. Gradually the picture builds up.

It is the same with well-being education more generally. Parents have a responsibility to teach discernment by reinforcing involvement in some pursuits and not others. The twin, related, cultures of fame and consumption may tempt children into misleading understandings of what makes a life go well. Parents do not *begin* by explaining why they are misleading; they simply keep the impact of these forces on their children as low as possible and engage them in other things. But they can begin to draw children into the downsides of celebrity and consumerism early on; and schools can continue their work in the direction of a deepening grasp of sociological, economic and ethical considerations.

On the road to intellectual autonomy, children need protection against those who try to impose on them a vision of how to live. Sometimes this is a peer group, perhaps acting as a conduit for the cultures just mentioned. Sometimes, families themselves can be similar conduits. At all events, there should be some way, within the school if not within the family, in which children can be encouraged to distance themselves from group pressures and form their own judgements about the good life. They need protection, too, against powerful institutions or individuals eager to proselytise their own ways forward.

The best protection is intellectual. Young people can learn to ask the right critical questions. 'Is A right in wanting me to do X?' 'What gives him or her the authority to lay down how one should live?' Some insight into the motives, psychodynamics and ways of operating of gurus and pied pipers is also useful. Literature and film can help. *The Prime of Miss Jean Brodie* is a classic film about a teacher in a girls' school who sets out to bind her 12-year-old pupils to her own philosophy of life. A more recent example is the German film *The Wave (Die Welle)*. In this, a secondary school teacher decides to get his class to see how totalitarianism can gain a hold – by setting himself up as the leader of a new cult into which he successfully – and disastrously – indoctrinates his students.

Viewing and discussing films like these can help to arm pupils against such domination, not only from charismatic teachers but also from self-appointed gurus elsewhere. Children need to make up their own minds about a fulfilling life and its constituents. It is not easy for them to do so. Most of them are unlikely to be prey to an individual *führer*. But all of them are daily exposed to unspoken messages their school as a whole reinforces about what things in life are worthwhile.

If the message is that no one has a privileged answer and that all of us are welcome to join the discussion, they are in good hands. But if everything a school does celebrates academic achievement and exam passing, without encouraging debate about this, it may well build up wider beliefs in its pupils from which some will find it hard to shake free. Some, not surprisingly, may get the idea that the highest form of life is contemplative or scholarly. This should raise no eyebrows if they choose this path, having explored alternatives. But if, day after day, the message seeps into their minds unawares, that is another story. Other students may be picking up a more instrumental perspective on life – that what is worth spending time on is what will produce goods further down the line: exam grades, three years of fun at university, hedge fund manager by 30 . . . Others, again, hearing only the school's one-track message, may let the media's louder beckonings towards fame, comfort, glamour and excitement drown it out.

Schools, then, should be attuned to the subliminal communications they send out about how one should live. Their top-down culture, if they still have it, should give way to something more fitting our democratic society. Human well-being is a slippery notion to get hold of; and young people need plenty of opportunities to think it through and discuss it with others.

Providing these should be a central task of the school. In this context, discussion is not merely a learning tool to help students see things more clearly. It might be used in that way in teaching geometry, say, but here its function is more subtle. Sharing one's thoughts and feelings is an inalienable feature of personal well-being, if not of doing mathematics. This is because here, as we saw earlier, there are no authorities, no experts to whom we can turn for correct answers. We are all able, in principle, to get inside the activities and relationships on which a flourishing life is founded; and we become better able, in the process, to participate in discussion about the endlessly open issues that this area brings with it.

Children are not in a position to reflect about a fulfilling life without extensive experience of its components. Their families have started them along the road; and it is a large part of the school's remit to take them further. This means a rethinking of its traditional role, excessively weighted as it has been towards academic and theoretical learning. Another thing the school can do, especially as pupils get older, is to begin to draw them into the cultural history of worthwhile pursuits, as sketched earlier in this chapter. This may well be of interest in its own right, but the intrinsic reason for getting inside this kind of history is entwined with another. It is this that I want to emphasise. It goes back to the issue of expertise about the nature of a flourishing life. Young people gaining these broader perspectives on what well-being is, and how the shape it takes is partly a product of our own history, are better placed to participate in ongoing reflection and discussion about it.

There are obvious implications here for citizenship education. What I have been describing is a part of students' induction into becoming democrats. They are being equipped as contributors to a conversation about human well-being taking place not only within national frontiers but, increasingly, on a global plane. Via face-to-face interactions at home and work, via internet and mobile, we may – with luck – be moving from a world where the media reinforce inadequate visions of a good life based on pleasure, fame and luxury towards a more democratic one in which we all, ideally, participate as informed insiders.

Chapter 12

Depth without spirituality?

1.

Are all worthwhile activities *equally* valuable? Or are some more worthwhile than others? I have said very little about this so far, apart from rejecting Mill's argument that the pleasures of the mind are of higher value than those of the body. It's time to look at the issues more squarely.

I was at a conference in Kofu, Japan, a few years ago. Not knowing the language, I skipped a number of sessions, and spent some of them wandering around the town. Once I found myself in a large building filled with several hundred patchinko machines, in front of each of which sat a man feeding in money or watching a little ball zig-zag downwards. I wondered whether these people came here on a regular basis. It certainly looked a serious business – more like a job of work than fun. The whole scene reminded me of the endless rows of office workers at their desks in Chaplin's *Modern Times*.

Is playing slot-machines a worthwhile activity? Let's imagine a case – which may or may not fit the patchinko men – where the players are not acting under the delusion that the chances of winning are high. Let's also take it that playing for its own sake is of major importance to them.

We could take a short way with this and simply deny that the activity is worthwhile – as I was tempted to do with the sand counter in Chapter 8. But this could be storing up trouble, for we might then be pressed on the criteria that let some things in and keep others out – and that might not be easy.

Need we assume, I wonder, that there *is* a line between worthwhile and non-worthwhile activities? Another way of looking at this is in terms of worthwhile *features*. Playing arcade machines can be fun to do with one's friends; it has elements of suspense; it has moments of joy when the coins cascade out of the kitty.

Perhaps we should say that playing slot-machines is *not much* of a worthwhile activity, rather than that it is not worthwhile at all. That, after all, is how people often treat it. It can be fun for half an hour, especially on a rainy seafront.

If we are looking for an activity that has *nothing at all* worthwhile about it, we would have probably have to fall back on imaginary cases. Someone who just adores standing alone for hours in a dark room thinking about nothing. Someone systematically making small incisions all over his flesh. If there's no further story to tell about religious practices or anything else that shows these activities have a point, they do indeed seem worthless.

I am aware that the account of well-being I've presented in the book may seem uninspiring. Pursuits with an element of profundity about them like the arts have been lumped in with more mundane things like playing football, weeding one's garden, watching soap operas, doing a minimally meaningful job. I've even been reluctant entirely to rule out mindless activities like playing slot-machines. Isn't it time to do more justice to differences in quality? If, as we would probably all agree, there are different degrees of worthwhileness, couldn't we now look into the depths rather than stay in the shallows?

Let's see how we go. The big question is: What *count* as 'the depths'. It is difficult to get very far along this road without coming across the word 'spirituality'. This has religious origins, but religiously minded people are the first to tell you that secular folk have a use for the term. Think of listening to Beethoven's last string quartets; watching a performance of *King Lear*; being in a long-term loving relationship; watching the sun setting over mountains. Such things can put us in touch with a deeper – or higher – part of our nature. We understand ourselves more fully.

It would be good if we could discuss these matters without using language that only gets in the way. If 'spirituality' boils down to self-understanding, let's stick with the vocabulary we know. The problem with 'spirituality' is that religious people tend to associate it with 'the human spirit' in a religious sense, that is, with the enduring part of us, our essential self that transcends mortal existence. When *they* say that listening to Beethoven puts them in touch with their deeper or higher self, it is often this transcendent entity that they have in mind. If we want a language with which secular people can feel comfortable, it is better to look elsewhere.

But before we do so, let's stay for a moment with the religious perspective on depth. This is still a potent cultural force, even in a society that finds religious claims increasingly hard to swallow. It tends to concentrate on one or more of the following areas: nature, the self, other people. There is a reason for this, in that each of them, it is held, can bring us face-to-face with the transcendent.

- Mountains, the curl of the surfer's big wave, a spring garden in blossom can be vivid witnesses to the heterogeneity of God's creation.
- Access to God can also come through the Self, given the intimate connection of the human soul with the divine consciousness. This may take the form of meditation, turning inwards, trying to get in touch with one's essential self.

- For some people, it may take the form of communion with other selves.

Not all of us live inside the religious framework that makes sense of things in this way. Yet many of us outside it still fall under its sway. As an agnostic from the cradle, I spent ages as a young man being some kind of Wordsworthian nature-worshipper, sensing the mystery of it all breathing through from hill-sides and sunlit streams. I was drawn, too, to texts on the mysteriousness of being in the world, endlessly self-interrogating and in quest of someone with whom our fused consciousness would lead to existence on a higher plane.

I was up, therefore, for mystery. Even much later in life, readier to discount the religious origins of these yearnings, I have found myself attracted to statements I have found in contemporary philosophy like 'the good life for man is the life spent in seeking for the good life for man' (MacIntyre, 1981: 204). The idea of a quest for what has until now lain hidden has been immensely appealing.

Suppose religion is eyewash. Is it possible to see through it entirely and yet retain the idea that some activities, not least those to do with nature, the self and others, possess a depth that sunbathing or watching snooker lack?

Nature

Take nature – as experienced directly, or indirectly through the arts. One source of our attachment to it is still religion, but in a non-believing context. We can enjoy Turner's seascapes and Wordsworth's descriptions of the Lake District affected by our knowledge that, for them, nature was a divine force. We can see and read their works as if we, too, were religious, even though we have put all that behind us. This empathetic perspective gives our enjoy-ment an extra layer. This comes on top of feelings and thoughts we may have of a wholly secular sort. These latter are themselves many-layered.

Thoughts closest to a religious perspective are about the brute existence of things at all. Dwelling on a particular, 'the meanest flower that blows' or an alpine glacier, can bring on cosmos-scoped wonder. This is heightened by the reflection that we, as human beings, are alone in our consciousness that we are experiencing this emotion. The difference from a religious attitude is that the wonder stops with wonder. If there is mystery, it is mystery strictly in the sense that there are things – like how it is there is anything at all – that we do not know. There is no belief in a being behind the appearances, a conscious presence, an object of veneration. Religious educators are fond of the phrase 'awe and wonder' when talking about the feelings they wish to evoke in their pupils, including non-religious children for whom *Religious education* is a compulsory subject. But the secular stops with wonder; 'awe' crosses the line.

Another secular attitude puts cosmic frissons to one side – at least consciously – and foregrounds only the particular and immediate. The robin keeping you anxiously in sight as it hops from tree to tree; the overnight eruption of a tree peony; pink blossom strewing the front path from a roadside tree... Nature is full of delights like these, intrinsic pleasures of perception.

Shall we group them with the intrinsic pleasures of playing fruit-machines? Are they at the shallow end of the depth continuum?

I don't think so. They take us beyond the world of isolated sensations, of self-contained experience. Whether by nature or through culture, probably both, we are fashioned to respond with joy to natural beauty. Although thoughts about the ephemeralness of our existence may not be in our focal awareness, they may well be background presences. They make us feel, as we say, 'glad to be alive', participants for this brief tract of consciousness in something literally wonderful.

The example gives us an indication of how 'depth' should be interpreted, once we have discarded religious myths. It shows that it is to be understood in terms of layered perspectives of understanding and emotion. What seems from one standpoint to touch only the surface of things – the sight of inch-long *cosmos* seedlings bending towards the sun on a window sill – can, from another, make contact with what is foundational to us.

The representation of nature in art adds further possibilities of value-layering. We see pigments, listen to words, enjoy the surface beauties of both. Our imagination presents us with sights, sounds, smells and tastes in our minds. The artist shapes these for us to evoke a certain mood, to heighten a narrative, to reflect profounder thoughts about human existence.

It is this complexity of values that makes for depth, that leads us back from the surface to the substructure, without crossing the line dividing this from an alleged transcendent.

Selves – one's own and others'

In the religious story, the human mind, one's own or another's, offers a glimpse of the eternal. Communion with oneself or with an intimate other, can put us in touch with the transcendent world.

In the story, the mind is a different kind of entity from the body. You can see the latter, but you can't see the mind. It is something inner, while our physical self is something outer. You may see me walking or breathing, but you cannot see me thinking. I live here behind an invisible wall and can keep myself to myself without your knowing. The mind is a private place. It is at the core of my and your existence. Fundamentally, as a non-mortal entity or soul, it is what we are.

Plenty, then, of mystery and depth here. If, that is, the story is true. But this is doubtful. When I see, hear, think, desire, feel pain, I am the subject of these states of consciousness, in the sense that it is *I* who see and hear etc. But that does not mean my mind is an entity. 'Subject' does not equate to 'substance'. Your dog can hear you when you call to her. It is *she* who hears. But this is far from saying that there is an invisible mental entity inside her skin.

Inside our own skins there is no non-material world to explore. If, in order to locate the essential me, I reflect on the fact that I am in some or other conscious state, the I that is doing the reflecting is not included in the I that I am reflecting on. If I try to pin it down by reflecting on this higher-order self, there is, once again, a reflecting I that is not at the same time an object of reflection. The search for this elusive self could clearly go on for ever. It is a philosopher's wild-goose chase.

I am not saying there's no mystery at all in this area. I cannot help but wonder at the fact that some organisms – very few, as far as we know, in the whole universe – are capable of conscious states – that dogs can hear whistles and eagles see their prey. It is equally an object of wonder that human beings, again perhaps alone in the cosmos, are capable not only of consciousness but also of self-consciousness in the sense of being aware of the conscious states they experience.

All this is indeed mysterious; in the sense, that is, that these are things we cannot, yet, explain. But *not* in the spooky sense of 'mystery' that leads us to look for answers in a transcendent world.

I'm not saying either that there is no possibility of depth in this area. To a large extent, the mental experiences of human and other animals connect them with the world outside themselves. Sight, hearing, smell, taste, desire pain, memory, are useful to us all in surviving in an often difficult or hostile environment. But because human beings are self-conscious as well as conscious creatures, it is possible for them to turn inwards as well as outwards and reflect on aspects of their own existence. Not only is this possible, it is also an essential element in living a flourishing life. Although I have said a lot about the place of worthwhile pursuits in the latter, it cannot, it seems, *just* consist in these. It is not parcelled without remainder into stretches of time devoted now to teaching literature, now to walking in the woods, now to cooking dinner, now to watching a Buster Keaton movie. A busy modern life may seem to approximate to this, but something, nevertheless, is left out of account. We also spend time reflecting on how our lives are going, both globally, in checking and reconsidering our priorities, reflecting on the wisdom of past decisions etc., and also in a more ongoing way, in responding to everyday vicissitudes. There may be some temptation to include such episodes of self-understanding as examples of yet another worthwhile activity to be added to our list. But that would be to undervalue and misconstrue the place of such reflection in personal well-being. It is not normally just another option – like walking in the woods or chatting to one's spouse – that may contribute to one person's well-being, but not another's. The pursuit of practical self-knowledge of this kind is essential to *everyone's* flourishing. In any case, it is not usually an activity into which one throws oneself with gusto, like watching a good film. There may be different degrees of immersion here in different people: some enjoy this kind of introspective activity more than others; but for all it is unavoidable.

Occasionally, the quest for self-knowledge is undertaken for intrinsic reasons. Say I'm retired and want to make sense of the 250 intimate journals that I wrote as a young man and are now in boxes in a corner of the cellar. I want to get inside the skin of this prolix young person who is now almost a stranger to me and who disclosed to himself so much of his everyday thinking in luxuriant Victorian prose. For the most part, however, self-understanding is a practical virtue that acts as a compass to keep us on life's road. I go further into this in Part 2.

We can say something partly along the same lines about communion with other people. Being in close, intimate, loving relationships is, for most people, the pivot of a fulfilling life. One of its many facets is exploring with the other how each of us thinks and feels about all sorts of matters. There are often practical reasons for this, but these are hard to untwine from intrinsic ones – perhaps harder than with the pursuit of self-knowledge on its own. For most of us, this kind of activity is immensely absorbing in itself.

There is no need to get all religious about the significance of the Other in linking us with the eternal. The aura that comes with that capital O is something to be dispelled. There is no need, either, to labour the many-layered quality possible in intimate conversation, especially between people who have known each other a long time. *This* is what gives it depth, not any alleged spirituality.

2.

The first part of this chapter has been mainly about a non-spiritual take on depth. Let's get back to the issue raised at its start, about whether all activities with any element of the intrinsically valuable about them are of equal worth. Is playing draughts as worthwhile as researching the history of Anglo-American relations? Are delivering milk and being prime minister on a par?

The issue reminds me of judgements about works of art. Is listening to the Beatles as aesthetically rewarding as listening to Mahler? Are Dickens's novels better than those of Scott Fitzgerald? In each case, are there sound criteria for grading items in a line from best to worst?

We should put snobbishness to one side. In the arts and in intellectual matters more generally, a distinction is often made between 'high' and 'popular' culture. Some people wouldn't dream of going to a pop concert, but attend operas at Glyndebourne. Someone else willingly curls up with Gibbon's *Decline and Fall* but would never watch a TV series on the beastlier Roman emperors. It is not hard to find similar spurnings and embracings in activities more generally – building up an aviary of rare birds, but not keeping pigeons; polo, not rugby league; wearing bespoke designer clothes, not dresses from Monsoon.

If the only basis for these kinds of gradings is to do with marking social superiority, we can ignore it. This is as true for the arts as for other activities. But is there any more solid reason for arranging artistic activities in a hierarchy of value?

Aestheticians are not, generally speaking, into league tables. They tend to be less interested in comparative judgements than in exploring and celebrating the variety of aesthetic values – generally, or as instantiated in particular works. It would be absurd to look for some way of ranking all art works in order. At the same time, it is *not* absurd to say that a painting by Rembrandt has all kinds of qualities not found in a typical portrait at a village art exhibition, or that *Dr Zhivago* is a better novel than a Mills and Boon.

But we have to be careful. The judgements just made have been (a) of the same type of artwork, and (b) of works at opposite ends of the scale. Where these conditions do not apply, comparisons of value are often more difficult, if not impossible. Is Velasquez's *Las Meninas* of higher aesthetic value than Milton's *Paradise Lost*? Is Lincoln Cathedral better than Exeter?

How well does this discussion of art illuminate the world of personal fulfilment? Here, too, there is more mileage in exploring the wealth and variety of worthwhile activities than in constructing hierarchies. Mill and others rate mental pleasures above physical ones. Walking in the country is a physical activity if anything is, and studying formal logic a mental one. But I see no reason why the first should be inferior to the second.

Even though hierarchies are hard to defend, there are reasons why some people tend to be drawn to more thickly textured pursuits. We have already discussed this in the aesthetic realm. Similar considerations apply in the broader field of personal goods. It is understandable why, for some people, certain activities have more attractive potential than others. For many of those acquainted with both, reading Goethe's poetry or being in a close relationship or teaching citizenship may have greater pulling power than playing draughts.

It is not that human beings are programmed to become bored with more simple activities and to move on to more complex ones. Many people would not be satisfied by more complex versions of the same thing – say a different type of draughts with complicated new rules. But they might well be drawn to something that opens up new horizons for them.

And this is what one finds in the magnet activities I described in the last-but-one paragraph. Reading Goethe is not simply a more complex activity than reading nursery rhymes. It opens a gate into worlds of new and already possessed but recollected values, and embroiderings on these. To call being in a close, longstanding, loving relationship more complex than being on speaking-and-greeting terms with one's neighbour is to miss the point. It incorporates so many forms of value. These can include shared sexual and other enjoyments, the opportunity to be fully open about one's feelings and thoughts, the joint creation of private spaces, support and succour, conversation and shared reflection on the finer texture of one's and others' lives, and much else besides. Some of these values can come via other routes than intimacy. What makes the latter a distinguishable value in itself is the particular way in which it encapsulates these.

It is not surprising that people are often drawn to activities that are ethically more many-layered in this way. This is not to imply that a line can be drawn between the many-layered and the non-many-layered. There is not a higher category and a lower one. We find, rather, all kinds of concatenations of values in different activities. This is a challenge to any attempt to regiment the value world into tidier categories.

For the same reason, it would be incorrect to identify more worthwhile activities with more thickly textured ones. Other things can be magnets too – simple pleasures like strolling around in the warm sunshine after a morning of rain. Is this of lower value than reading *On The Origin of Species*?

A final thought on depth. It takes time to build up many-layered involvement. A first acquaintance with a work of great art, like the beginnings of a love affair, brings its own enchantment. But deeper sources of fulfilment in these areas are built up slowly. The same is true of other intrinsically worthwhile activities, not least forms of meaningful work.

This is not to say that you can't flourish unless your life is full of enduring commitments. It is not an argument in favour of lifelong marriage or never changing your job or sticking with the same leisure pursuits.

Issues for education

Along with 'breadth', 'depth' has been a desideratum of the traditional school curriculum, but, like its twin, has been conceived in too narrow a fashion. 'Breadth' has usually referred to coverage of all the main forms of knowledge, and 'depth' to specialised learning within them. But once we think of education as handmaiden of well-being rather than aide to the academy, the scene changes. 'Breadth' has to do with the historically developing array of well-being pursuits described in the last chapter; 'depth' with the layered perspectives of understanding and emotion within these, described earlier in this one.

In education for well-being, learners are introduced to both breadth and depth. This begins to happen very early in their upbringing. For the child of a few months, personal relationships centre around the comforts and pleasures provided by immediate family members. By 3, the child has become used to interacting, in subtly differentiated ways, with grandparents, friends of the family and their children, friends and teachers from nursery, relatives abroad via Skype, regular visitors to the house, people in shops, characters on television and DVD. Over the same period, he is coming to appreciate more of the initially hidden delights of social intercourse: playing with toys together, receiving and giving affection and recognition, joining in work around the house and garden, being read to, finding things funny.

I have been talking about relationships education, but similar stories could be told, even by age 3, about, for instance, his widening and deepening acquaintance with the arts – music, song, stories, film, pictures.

Seeing that all this happens by the age of 3, how much further development there can be on both dimensions by 18! If we concentrate now on depth, it is a pity that schools do not do more to build on the developing interests that children have. This is standard practice in any good home, but hit-and-miss when it comes to formal education. I mentioned in the last chapter my own Dickens-fest before going to grammar school and failure to read anything after I got there. There are a million other such experiences that others could relate. In many cases, I suspect, the school is unaware of these enthusiasms.

How could things be done better? In several ways. There should be some kind of regular system whereby every child's particular passions are made known to the school. Time could be carved out of the school day in which children can pursue this passion further, singly or in groups, and under appropriate supervision. These interests, together with progress made in them, should be recorded, with monitoring and changes of teacher in mind.

I am assuming here activities to be pursued at deeper and deeper levels of profundity. Getting further into types of road vehicle is not good enough on its own. But it still has promise that an imaginative adult can exploit. She can lead the child back in time, to a world without cars and lorries; develop his interest in roads, traffic lights, bypasses, motorways towards insight into the problems of organising whole traffic systems. She is unlikely to be an expert in the area but can encourage him to find out more from library books and the internet, motivating him at the same time to make progress in reading and investigative skills.

Any interest that a child is likely to have is capable of deeper development in this way. It is no accident that the examples just given move in the direction of human interests – changes in culture, basic needs, conflicts of value between road users and others. For human concerns, including the structures of value lying behind them, provide an arena of many-layered interest to which all of us constantly turn and return, not only directly, through our relationships and other interactions, but also imaginatively, via literature and other arts, and more analytically, via history, philosophy and other humanistic pursuits.

Visual arts, including film, and, especially, literature are, educationally, of particular importance, because of their deliberately seductive powers. It is the artist's, especially the writer's, task to seize our attention at the level of immediate incident and sensuous experience, and to lead us from there into hidden realms of thought and feeling. The experience is both enjoyable in itself and also a symbolic reminder, usually at a subconscious level, of the journeys from surface to depth we make in so many other of our activities and relationships.

In this way, a good artist is an educator. Practically speaking, in the world of scarce educational resources, this is a bonus. Provided the learner can read well enough to benefit from a book or other work of this sort, formal teaching has less of a role. A novelist or other storyteller can be a great – and inexpensive – teaching assistant.

I do not want to overdo matters connected with human life. There are layers beyond layers, too, in mathematics and in the physical sciences, and in listening to and playing music. Some children find an early fulfilment in areas like these. Whatever his or her passion, each child needs space and time to take it further.

At the same time, deep immersion in mathematics or the sciences *alone* could well fail to realise the good I am trying to articulate. If pupils found themselves travelling further and further into a self-contained world, with no links at all to wider human concerns, they could be missing out on so much. Few such, fortunately, are as sealed off in other areas of their lives. Their relationships, perhaps their interest in politics or the arts, enmesh them in deeper human concerns. So does the self-knowledge they need to pilot their own way through life.

And yet we all know, or know of, people locked inside some technical specialism, perhaps in commerce or industry, who have meagre outside interests or connections, and yet seem to find their single-track life all they could desire. Are they leading a fulfilling life? They meet many of the criteria I have suggested for this. Assuming we are not into either/or thinking, we could reasonably call their lives flourishing to some extent.

Yet it may be that what they are lacking in their lives is not, as it were, just one further layer of satisfaction, but something which, for the rest of us, makes all the difference between what would be, for us, a thin, virtually wasted, life and a genuinely fulfilling one. I have in mind keeping in touch with such elemental features of our common human nature as our capacity for intimacy; self-awareness; brevity of life; intellectual, imaginative and other powers; and irresolvable conflicts among our ethical ideals and values.

That is why schools have to be so wary of steering children too blinkeredly in some specialist direction, and why the arts and humanities are not just other curriculum territories alongside, and on a par with, mathematics and the sciences, but at the very centre of a worthwhile education.

With this qualification, I come back to my earlier point that schools should provide space and time for children to pursue their passions, whether for the sciences or for something else. You may think I am rooting for an earlier introduction of the option system that English secondary schools provide for students over 14. There is certainly a similarity. In both cases, children do what they want, rather than have, to do. But there is one big difference. In my proposal, the main motive that drives children onwards is *love* – an all-absorbing delight in their chosen object of interest. Post-14 option work is far more under the sway of fear and hope. It is not lost in the present but is future-orientated, towards a good performance in public examinations, with all their life-shaping implications. How much better is the way of love! Teenage years would no longer be in thrall to a system that generates so much public competitiveness and so much private grief.

Is this realistic? Could we diminish the power of examinations? If the will is there, easily. The record of interests and achievements suggested for younger children could, without difficulty, be continued throughout their school career. If, collectively, we only had the will, we could find ways of making it attractive to the institutions that now rely on exam results.

Willing is hard, because the examination system has been such a staple feature of traditional schooling. The chain from (a) a broad subject-based curriculum, to (b) public examinations in these subjects, to (c) higher education and professional jobs, has governed secondary education in Britain and elsewhere for 150 years and more. But there is no reason why the system should go on for ever. This book proposes radical change at all three junctures: a well-being-based curriculum; ongoing records of achievement; remodelled universities and employment arrangements. There is more on the last of these in Part 2.

Back to 'depth'. I have been arguing for giving learners more space to penetrate the less-visible layers of their passions, but I wouldn't want all their schooling to be dominated by this, any more than I would want the whole of a flourishing human life to be taken up with exploring its deeper strata. As hinted earlier, simpler pleasures – delight in the surface beauty of the world, enjoying light-hearted banter, looking forward to a favourite soap – are not necessarily lower in some hierarchy of value. Would I have done better as a self-fulfiller if I had not spent yesterday evening watching a DVD of James Cagney in *The Roaring Twenties*, but had instead read *Macbeth*?

I have said little in this section about 'spiritual development'. This was one aim of the National Curriculum in 1988 and still informs it. In a religious context, it implies progression towards the invisible world of eternal spirit. I hope I have said enough to distinguish it from the very different kind of penetration of the invisible described above.

Chapter 13

The meaning of life

The last chapter was about depth. We come finally to what for some people is the deepest question of all: 'What is the meaning of life?'

When you or I review the meaningfulness or meaninglessness of our own life, can we divorce this from the question of whether it fits into any wider framework of purposes?

Our religious inheritance, Muslim, Jewish as well as Christian, tells us it does. Human life is part of God's creation. It exists for a reason, a reason in God's mind. The meaningfulness of any individual's life is a function of the meaningfulness of human life in general.

What am I living for? What is my purpose in the world? Questions that made sense in a religious context are rejected by the non-believer because of the assumption, embedded in them, that there is something extrinsic to my life that gives it point. But nothing like this exists. I live; I die; end of story.

This seems to make my being on Earth pretty meaningless. What is a human life, after all? A few years of days spent breathing, eating, fornicating, thinking, working, sleeping, and that's it. A micro-speck in a godless universe, and then not even that.

When I was very young, I was much affected by this way of thinking, courtesy of then fashionable existentialist writings. I would stand looking for ages at a clump of cow parsley, sunsets, a night full of stars, thrilling both at their alienness and at my consciousness of them, the latter soon to be switched off.

It's hard to know what to make of all this. When I think now of my present confrontations with the universe, they do indeed appear, literally, wonderful. But this reaction is separable from the sense of absurdity that used to accompany it.

For belief in the meaninglessness of life is only intelligible as a flipside of the religious belief that life is meaningful. It depends on a religious framework to make sense. An enchanted universe, full of unseen spirits and hidden significances in ordinary events, turns into an empty one. The extrinsic reason why human life exists has fallen away, leaving it without point.

Is there any alternative? Can we get away from meaninglessness without being re-ensnared by the old religious myths?

Francis Galton, H. G.Wells and other eugenicists thought we could, since there *is* a purpose to our lives, a higher state of evolved being. So did other believers in inevitable human progress, Marxists and others. So did, and do, those, myself at times included, who have been troubled by life's absurdity and gone in quest of the key to unlock its secret.

Where to look for it? Somewhere in the Himalayas, perhaps, among lamas, maharishis and prayer wheels? If we only meditate hard enough, free our minds of everything except the One, transcend the desiring Self, will we discover the still point at which everything forms up into an intelligible whole?

Or is the key eating chickpeas and sourdough bread? Or taking mescalin? Or minutely controlling the rhythm of your breathing? In my younger, questing days, I always carried around a paperback called *The Culture of the Abdomen* for a regimen like this. I don't remember now whether it gave me what I was looking for.

Or is Gaia the answer? Are we all parts of a complex, living and non-living system that operates as a single organism?

The difficulty with all such solutions is that they are all still under God's shadow. They are ways of discovering significance in a world that seems meaningless. But if the descent into meaninglessness is only intelligible in the light of the old religious world-picture, so is the desperate attempt to escape from it.

In any case, aren't most of our lives meaningful enough already without having to find a hidden ingredient that will make them so? Think of the way most of us get on with day-to-day living, taking Jacob to the childminder, catching the bus into work, checking overnight emails, attending to customers, collecting Jacob, watching the new DVD of *Up In the Air* over a pizza. What makes our life meaningful is that it has a certain patterning to it. The activities and experiences that compose it are connected together in chains of connected purposes, subordinate ones nested within those of more central significance to us.

We don't depend on an umbilical connection to the universe to make sense of our lives. All we need is engagement in activities like these. As the philosopher Bernard Williams (1976: 209) has said, 'One good testimony to one's existence having a point is that the question of its point does not arise.' We simply get on with things.

That still leaves room for the *sense* that life is meaningless, perhaps even for its *being* meaningless. Think of the feelings of hopelessness that people experience when depressed or contemplating suicide. Perhaps they have lost a child or a partner or a homeland. The bottom has dropped out of their world. They see no point in carrying on. Their usual pattern of activities now means nothing to them.

This sort of meaninglessness is not a built-in feature of human life in general. It is a pathological notion, cropping up where the taken-for-granted intelligibility of normal life breaks down. It is very different from an existential sense of futility. It does not, above all, depend on a previous religious framework. It is not a reverse image of this.

Likewise, the meaningfulness of our everyday lives is not the product of a quest, a scramble out of the pit of absurdity. We do not *seek* meaning in our lives; we find it everywhere.

In all this talk of meaningfulness, have I drifted away from our main topic, personal fulfilment? Has fascination with religion's legacy led me astray?

Not really. Whatever else a flourishing life might be, it must at least make sense – in the anodyne sense of 'sense' I have just been using. A depressed or shattered existence that gives rise to feelings of pointlessness is not a thriving one. So meaningfulness *is* intimately related to flourishing. It is a necessary condition of it.

But it's not sufficient. Imagine someone whose life is full of misfortunes. Not meaning-threatening ones like being driven from one's home and homeland by an invader, but serious-enough ones like scarcely ever having enough money even for necessities, going deaf, being mugged or burgled, losing job after job, girl after girl. You would hardly call his a thriving life. Yet there is a structure to it. The man has, like the rest of us, all sorts of goals, works out ways of achieving them and overcoming obstacles. The only thing is that, *unlike* most of us, he has had an unbelievable amount of bad luck and has made endless bad judgements. His life is meaningful, no question. He never falls into despair so deep that he can't see the point of carrying on. He muddles along, forever hoping that things may get better. His life is meaningful, but far from fulfilling.

What more, then, needs to be added to its meaningfulness for a life to be flourishing? From the example given, it looks as if success rather than failure may have a lot to do with it. Here we come back to the features of well-being picked out in earlier chapters.

Issues for education

Where does the meaning of life appear in the English school curriculum? The only officially mentioned place is the *Religious education* curriculum. We are told that 'RE provokes challenging questions about the ultimate meaning and purpose of life'.

This appears to take it as read that life *has* an 'ultimate meaning and purpose'. The RE regulations fail to make the distinction discussed above between the 'meaningfulness' of life (a) as implying an external purpose, and (b) in its secular sense.

They do not *insist* that questions about meaning and purpose be looked at from a non-religious perspective. A 'secular world-view' *may* be included in RE lessons for 11–14-year-olds '*where appropriate*'. On the other hand, Christianity and at least two other principal religions *must* be studied.

Children might easily be led to think, therefore, that life has an extrinsic purpose, and never question this. There are implications here for their intellectual autonomy and hence their well-being. The issue is exacerbated in those faith schools in England, and some evangelical schools in America, where creationism is taught and Darwinian perspectives are excluded.

On the creationism/Darwinism issue more generally, it was only in 2009 that the British government decided to make the study of evolution compulsory in English primary schools, only to withdraw this requirement a year later. I mentioned in Chapter 2 the new emphasis on 'big ideas' in the English school curriculum. It is hard to think of a bigger idea from the last three centuries than evolution by natural selection. Why, then, exclude it?

Learning about evolution is a good way of enabling children to reflect on and challenge the very different message they may well be getting from their RE lessons, that human life has 'an ultimate meaning and purpose'. It is true that the two ideas do not contradict each other head on, since one can accept the Darwinian, non-purposive, account of why we are here, but still hold that God has put the Darwinian mechanisms in place for some further purpose of his own. This may be too sophisticated an idea for younger children, although there are good reasons why older students should take it on board. This aside, children should be acquainted, even at primary school, *both* with the idea that human life has been created for a divine purpose, *and* with the idea that it has come to be what it is through myriad contingencies in the story of natural selection. They should at least be equipped to entertain the idea that life may be meaningless in the traditional, religious sense.

If their school provides them with a well-being-based education on the lines explored in earlier chapters, there is little danger that they will think their life meaningless in the secular sense. They will usually be too caught up in absorbing, enjoyable activities and relationships to ask themselves whether their life makes sense.

*   *   *

These brief remarks bring us to the end of Part 1. Through its last dozen chapters, this has turned the concept of well-being this way and that, bringing facet after facet of it up to the light, so that we can grasp it in all its complexity. The point of this has been to give teachers and others involved in education a firmer hold on a central value informing their work, and to show how schools can embody it in their aims and practices. Since these educational applications have been scattered across the 12 chapters, I need now to bring them together. I do this in Part 2.

Part 2

Education for well-being: the way forward

In Part 2, I enlarge on points made in Part 1 in presenting a more unified argument about education for well-being. This falls into four chapters, of which the first two are the shortest. Chapter 14 reminds us of philosophical claims already made about the concept of well-being, while Chapter 15 explores wider social changes needed if education for well-being is to be more than a pipe dream. Chapter 16 looks at the aims of a well-being-orientated education, and Chapter 17 at ways in which schools, in particular, can seek to realise them.

Chapter 14

What well-being is: a summary

'Education, education, education!' Tony Blair's famous electoral pledge in 1997 sounds, in retrospect, like promising more of what we had already. What he *should* have called for is a different conception of education – one that aims at the promotion of well-being, the child's and other people's. I will say more about this in a moment. First, I will pull together the conceptual points I have been making about well-being.

A flourishing life is one filled with successful and whole-hearted engagement in worthwhile activities and relationships. It has to be, on the whole, *successful*, since repeated failure in our projects and liaisons clearly detracts from our well-being. It has to be *whole-hearted* because, again, it is hard to see how dragging ourselves through even the most valuable pursuits in a tired, listless, merely dutiful or uncommitted way can make our life go well. What counts as *worthwhile* is partly dependent on our biology: we would not prize sexual intimacy if we reproduced, amoeba-like, by fission. But it is mainly a cultural matter. In Britain and other countries, we are heirs to a remarkable efflorescence, especially over the last few centuries, in new forms of art, personal relationships, public service and other occupations, as well as hosts of further activities that add richness to our lives. Although these are culturally determined, in that if it were not for the history of the last 400 years we may now well be without them, they are not culturally relative. Bach's music may have been the product of a Protestant devotional world, but its aesthetic power has not diminished as that world has been left behind.

There are no final authorities on worthwhileness and hence on the flourishing life. There are gurus galore who will tell you how best to live, but part of any young person's education will include acquiring a judicious scepticism towards them all. At the same time, the individual has more than his or her own hunches and gut feelings to rely on. What was open only to the seriously wealthy in the past now belongs to millions. Think of listening to music, travelling abroad, reading novels, bringing up a family in some comfort. There are no final authorities on well-being, but there are now countless numbers of us who not only, on the basis of experience, share some kind of consensus about what makes life worth living, but also participate in on-going discussion on the topic. It should be a social policy objective to see our numbers swell further. One aspect of democratic citizenship is an interest in what makes for a flourishing life; it is central to large political questions about the kind of society we wish to bring about.

Some worthwhile activities and relationships have more to them than others. While there is no sharp dividing line between 'higher' and 'lower' pursuits, contrasting, for instance, the 'pleasures of the mind' with the 'pleasures of the body', there are undeniable differences in depth. Sometimes this is put in terms of spirituality, but it is better to avoid this expression with all its misleading associations and to think more archaeologically, in terms of reaching deeper layers of appreciation and feeling. We see this *par excellence* in personal relationships and in the arts, but it is also a feature of other aspects of our lives like jobs and free-time interests. For most of us, if we are to live fulfillingly, we cannot pursue *all* our activities, however worthwhile, in a narrow, self-contained way. Most of them are constantly reconnecting us, in their deeper reaches, with basic elements of our shared human nature.

Human beings can lead flourishing lives in all kinds of societies. There is even good reason for applying the concept, in some reduced form, to other animals. In a liberal-democratic society like our own, the concept we use reflects the fact that nearly everyone is expected to choose for themselves the pursuits they wish to follow, rather than leaving this to custom or authority. Personal autonomy thus becomes a major well-being value in its own right. It brings its own burdens, in that we often face difficult choices between this or that consideration.

There are certain prerequisites of flourishing. These include biological needs to do with food, air, water and health; and social needs like income, education, recognition and free time. In a liberal-democratic society, liberty of thought and action is a necessary condition of autonomous well-being. Good fortune can also be counted a basic need, as can the personal qualities we need for flourishing. These dispositions range from managing our bodily desires and emotions to intelligently adapting the means we follow in pursuit of our ends, coping with setbacks, co-operativeness, and many others.

Several misconceptions need defusing. A flourishing life is not to be identified with a pleasurable one, or with a life in which one succeeds in satisfying one's major informed desires. This casts doubt on links often made between well-being and wealth, celebrity or positional goods. Secondly, in order to flourish, we do not need to have our own flourishing as a goal. This may indeed be counter-productive. There are also problems with the belief that leading a flourishing life requires planning, in broad outline, what shape that life will have. This suits some, but others live more spontaneously and thrive just as well.

The familiar contrast between personal well-being and morality or altruism is also misconceived. Doing what is morally right or seems to benefit others at one's own expense can often enhance our own well-being even if we have not intended this. Apart from this, so many of the pursuits that contribute to a person's own good have goals shared with others. This is true both of relationships and of co-operative activities. This makes it hard or impossible to disentangle what is good for oneself from what is good for others. None of this means that personal benefit cannot be immoral or at the cost of others' good; but it should be among the goals of a democratic community to encourage its citizens to adopt a conception of their own well-being that brings maximal overlap with others'.

Finally, it would be wrong to associate personal well-being too closely, as some do, with what one does in one's 'leisure'. Paid employment often involves whole-hearted engagement in a worthwhile activity. Think of a teacher or doctor who really loves their job. But many forms of paid work do *not* pass this bar. As heteronomous rather than autonomous activities, they are something which, income aside, one would rather be without. They take up a lot of time that could otherwise have been spent on something more fulfilling, and can be physically or mentally painful and exhausting into the bargain. There is a strong case, in a well-being society, for reducing the burdens of heteronomous work.

Chapter 15

Well-being for all in a more equal society

In Chapter 16, I shall be pulling together points made in Part 1 about educa-tion for well-being. But so much of the discussion there called for wider changes in society that it is best to begin with those. My focus is Britain, but the recommendations apply more broadly.

If schools are to play their part in promoting well-being *for all*, this only makes sense if the wider society also makes this a priority. In the mid-twentieth century, it did so. The post-1945 British 'welfare state' helped to reduce the poverty, bad housing, insecurity, ignorance and poor health that had blighted the prospects of the worse-off. Economic developments in the same period also benefited this group as well as others, leading both to improvements in working conditions and opportunities, and also to the reduction of domestic chores through labour-saving devices.

But the last two decades of the century saw well-being for all sidelined as a political objective. Although the Labour government of 1997–2010 did much to reverse this, at the end of this period, the UK, along with the USA and Portugal, was still among the three most unequal countries in the developed world in terms of income. Like the USA, it was also higher than countries more equal in rates of mental illness, illegal drug use, infant mortal-ity, general and child obesity, teenage births, children's experience of fighting, bullying and other forms of conflict, imprisonment, health and social problems, and working hours.

Britain is also lower than the same countries in life expectancy and social mobility. There is now a ten-year gap between the average age of male deaths in a northern town like Blackpool (73.6 years) and that in the rich London Borough of Kensington and Chelsea (84.3 years). Recent research by the Sutton Trust shows that life chances for the poorest quarter of the population born between 1958 and 1970 actually decreased.

There is plainly some way to go in enabling the whole UK population, and not just a fortunate section of it, to enjoy a flourishing life. If the authors of *The Spirit Level*, from which some of the above statistics come, are right in their analysis, decreasing income inequality holds the key, since more equal societies also tend to produce better results on all these other dimensions (Wilkinson and Pickett, 2010).

The more unequal the society, the more likely are misconceptions about the nature of well-being; the view, for instance, that associates it with success rather than failure, conventionally understood. From this perspective, well-being is necessarily a competitive good; it has to do with being singled out from those 'below' one in terms of greater income, 'better' education and more congenial work. It puts a premium on the possession of positional goods, with the likelihood that others will feel less worthy in lacking them.

The UK has historical obstacles to overcome if it is to resume its post-war impetus towards a more equal society. Deep in the shadows is a salvationist way of thinking about human well-being, prone to divide people into those marked out for success and the rest. Connected with this is a class system known for its tenacity. If the obstacles are to be surmounted, we need a narrowing of differentials in wealth and income as well as changes in attitude towards perceived social status and seeing life competitively as a zero-sum game. Changes in our schools can help here, not least as regards attitude change. I will come back to these.

Meanwhile, a comment about work. In the shadows lies the Protestant ethic of hard work as good for the soul. You find plenty of better-off people willing to work long hours at a job that they enjoy: in academia, school teaching, the media, medicine. The more heteronomous the job, the more likely it is to be associated with lower social status and, often, lower self-esteem. People less well-off do not often willingly choose their long hours of road-mending, working in a call centre or rubbish collection as part of a vision of the good life.

The other day I was with my little grandson in Sainsbury's car park. He was riveted by the work that four men were doing in a fenced-off area, collecting a tarry substance in a wheelbarrow, spreading it, rolling it and moving on to the next patch. One of the men, perhaps in his fifties, called out to me, 'Tell him to work hard at school; then he won't end up like us'.

If our watchword really is 'well-being *for all*', we have to challenge the belief that hard, time-consuming work of *any* kind is a virtue in itself.

There is a strong case for reducing the burden of heteronomous work falling on some individuals but not others. This should be a policy priority. Continuing economic growth has until recently been taken for granted as a good thing. There is no need to labour its threat to global sustainability, or its generation of goods and services that add little, if anything, to our well-being. We need to rethink what is really important in life. Reducing long hours of unwelcome work is *plainly* more worthwhile than enabling people to buy cars for others to envy. If we all had more of a sense of how one person's perceived advantage can mean another person's misfortune, we should be in a better position to move forward.

A specific way of doing so is suggested in the pamphlet *21 Hours*, published by the New Economics Foundation in 2010 (http://www.neweconomics.org/publications/21-hours). This proposes the gradual shortening of what is considered a 'normal' working week, from the present 40 hours or more to 21 hours. It gives us a practical guide to how the change could take place, its benefits, obstacles in its way and how they might be overcome. As it points out, and as we saw in the Introduction, Keynes envisaged a working week of 15 hours by 2030. Although he was out in his forecast, his belief that a shorter week would be enough to meet our satisfying material needs and to enable us to focus on 'how to use freedom from pressing economic cares', is very much in line with NEF ideas. Among other things, these foreground benefits to individual well-being, including a more fulfilling family life.

One reason why work is irksome for so many has to do less with hours than with autonomy. With paid work taking up 40 hours per week or more, it can make a difference to people's well-being how much control they have over what they do, and when and how they do it. Again, it is usually in less-desired, lower-paid jobs that we find the greatest constraints. Worker participation schemes, as in the John Lewis Partnership, are an obvious way forward. But they cannot overcome on their own the problem that people need more time, in the short lives they have, to spend on pursuits more fulfilling than checking home orders in some back office or checking out purchases at tills. Overall work reduction that provides everyone with an adequate and fairly distributed income must be a high priority.

Imagine a society restructured on these lines, with greater income equality, less in thrall to the work ethic and enabling more people to lead more of a fulfilling life. This has implications for education. In a society in which your chances of such a life are tied, as they are now, to the kind of job you do and your place in a social hierarchy of wealth and respect, one can well understand why parents pull out all the stops to secure a good academic education for their children, one that will lead on to a university degree and a nice job. Where less hangs on the kind of job you do, the less pressure there is likely to be to use schools and universities instrumentally in this way. They will be freer to concentrate more on absorbing, worthwhile activities, with less thought about competitive advantages.

In this new social vision, there will be less reason to tie universities as tightly as they are now tied to the full-time education of older teenagers. It has been taken as read for centuries that higher education studies should be end-on to school. This was understandable in an age when life expectancy was low. But a society built around well-being for all, its members likely to live into their eighties or beyond, has less reason to persist with old patterns.

It conceives post-school education in a different way. It rejects the myth that a university is some kind of privileged institution, set apart from, and above, other places like technical or further education colleges (White, 2009). The distinction between a university and a college is less a conceptual than a merely administrative one, its function being to maintain a conventional hierarchy.

The new society will create a unified, undifferentiated system of post-school colleges. These will no longer cater almost exclusively for older adolescents, with a tiny accretion of adult classes for other people. Campuses will be filled with persons of all ages, interested in part- or full-time pursuit of worthwhile practical, academic and aesthetic activities of their own choice.

This is not to rule out provision for those 18-year-olds who wish to pursue their studies straight after school. But there need not be the conventional pressures on them, as there are now, to do so full-time. As many young people are doing now at the Open University, they could take on part-time university studies after leaving school while holding down a job. Fiscal and other incentives could be devised to encourage them to consider later learning. (I think here of my own higher education. This began in earnest with a no-nonsense, part-time, evening-based degree at Birkbeck College, London, gained at the age of 30 – which helped to make up for three wasted years of full-time drift at Brasenose College, Oxford.)

Although some 18–20-year-olds will still be around as full-time students – and steps will be necessary to ensure that these are not mainly from more privileged backgrounds – most younger people will be in some sort of work. If this is for less than the current working week, it will leave them plenty of time for other things. Those studying part-time may be given special incentives to do so in the form of money and/or time.

This kind of pattern will break the stranglehold that universities have over secondary schools, shaping their curricula and forcing teachers and students to see what they are doing as bitter competition for a place in the social sun. This year, 2010, has seen how damaging this can be to people's well-being. More school students than ever before have achieved glittering A-level results, and as a consequence, more students than ever before have been denied a university place. The future, discounting the current recession, looks just as dark: greater numbers screwing up their intellects and powers of determination until they nearly snap; greater numbers opening their fateful envelope in August and seeing their years of labour become dust.

This is a crazy way to proceed. We could make the later years of secondary school so much more fulfilling for everyone if we changed tack. There will be resistance. The image of those three or four sparkling undergraduate years is a feature of our culture – as an aspiration for lower classes and an expectation for upper – 'the best years of one's life' – a time of freedom, of exploration, of responsible self-management, of discovering who one is.

If this is all so good for those who experience it, how fair is it that *they* should be enjoying it while *other* 19-year-olds are hard at work for pittances? As things are now, older school students not unnaturally see the prospect of three or four years of relative autonomy at college as a fair reward for all the years of slog for public examinations. 'It's like being on holiday every day of the week,' says the Sheffield University aerospace engineering student at the end of his first year. If we think the freedoms of university life a good thing, why not arrange things so that *every* young person has a self-discovering sabbatical?

This may seem too fanciful. It is in any case detachable from the more important message – that cutting out this last escalator in one's upward progress through the education system could bring such benefits to schools. Imagine them freed, post-14, from the shackles of public examinations! So much less reason for good teachers to prostitute themselves by teaching candidates how to play the system. So much more scope for students to throw themselves into studies and practical activities that grab them. Think of the horizons that often open up at adolescence: new passions, not only for relationships, but for the arts, philosophy and religion, a better world ... As things are now, so much of this has to be reined back for the sake of a clutch of good GCSEs or an A* in geography. Keeping teenage noses to the grindstone may be good for initiating youngsters into the work ethic and its rewards, but benefits for personal fulfilment are harder to see.

In this chapter I have outlined some of the changes needed in wider society if schools are to do more to help each pupil to enjoy a flourishing life. I am aware that these cannot take place overnight. But we can at least start to get things moving – there is no point in carrying on as we are.

Chapter 16

Education for well-being: the wider picture

Priorities

New society, new schooling. If we want a society built around well-being for all, we need schools that prepare people for this. I say more below about their relationships to families, about their well-being aims, about their learning arrangements. Before that, a question about priorities.

Just how *central* an aim should universal well-being be? It is, after all, not the only candidate. Supporting the economy is another. So is preparation for citizenship. There are others, too, if only in the shadows. Social selection, for example.

It is hard to think of *any* aim, actual or ideal, without *some* link to personal well-being. Economic goals are not ends in themselves; their point is to help people to lead more flourishing lives. The same goes for being a good citizen.

For some people, more intrinsic aims of education may seem counter-examples. I am thinking of such things as 'a love of learning for its own sake', or the aim cherished by Schools Minister Nick Gibb, and taken from Matthew Arnold: 'introducing children to "the best that has been thought and said" '.

Very often, as with Nick Gibb, this kind of aim accompanies a tough-minded insistence on academic subjects and a hard line towards personal and social learning. But this position is unstable. *Why* introduce children to the best literature, history, science or mathematics unless this is in some way *personally beneficial* to themselves or to others?

Admittedly, the main thrust of this book has been towards the child's own well-being, while some of the aims just mentioned are about more general welfare. This provokes the thought: since the child is a part of larger collectives, why don't we go straight for the bigger picture and aim only at the well-being of all?

We have to be careful. If schools are servants only of the general good, then depending on whether the parameters are national or global, each individual pupil's welfare counts for no more than one sixty-millionth part, or ten-billionth part, of the whole. In other words, it counts for virtually nothing at all. Sacrificing it completely for the sake of the totality is a hair's breadth away.

I'll take it we are ruling out this kind of utilitarianism. Under the banner of 'well-being for all', we are interested in what schools can do to help *each pupil* to lead a fulfilling life, not in using individuals merely as means to something else. But how shall we conceive this? Is the pupil's well-being to be our *only* consideration? Is it something untrumpable by other aims?

This book is not a treatise on the aims of education in general. But suppose we allow that some, at least, of the aims just mentioned must be accommodated. True, if *everyone's* well-being is *equally* important, social selection is an iffy one. But economic and moral/civic aims need not face this problem of privilege. What priority *vis-à-vis* them, if any, should personal well-being aims have?

Points made earlier should make us wary of treating these as separate from them. On the economic side, the work I do for a living gives me the money I need to lead a fulfilling life, and, if I whole-heartedly enjoy it, has intrinsic benefits as well. As for the moral/civic dimension, doing things to help other people can be, and normally is, a part of any individual's own flourishing.

Does this mean that the *only* aim that educators – parents as well as teachers – should follow is preparation for personal well-being? Should they direct all their energies towards helping each pupil to live flourishingly?

Provided that they are bringing children up within a generous-enough conception of their own good, this seems reasonable. If they were to draw a sharp line between self-interest and altruism, it would be hard to sustain. But I am assuming here that they will be encouraging children to have friendly, kindly, concerned relationships with those close to them, *and* to enjoy these as benefiting themselves. In less-intimate relationships, the same point applies. I am assuming children will see others' well-being in their local, national and global communities as inextricably related to their own. I am taking it, too, that they will want to do useful and absorbing work within the economy, again as an intrinsic and not merely instrumental element in their own well-being.

I must be careful not to claim too much. Human life is not a conflict-free zone, where interests always harmonise and never clash. Twice-weekly fish barbecues for friends and family drive neighbours from their gardens. However we try to square things, we all need to acquire considerateness and other familiar moral virtues. True, if we could get the fish-fryer to see the well-being of the next-door couple as in some way united with his own, the conflict could become not inter-, but intra-personal – like being torn between going for a walk or reading a novel. But to play safe, it is best to stop some way short claiming that the *only* thing the school should be doing is furthering the child's well-being.

One last thought. It would be possible for someone to accept everything

I have said, and yet favour a privileged education for some and a second-rate education for the rest. Each child's good is important, on this view, but some children's good has more to it than others'.

Majority School keeps children's flourishing centrally in its sights. It engages them in absorbing activities, extends their cognitive horizons, weaves in work preparation and civic goals and underlines the centrality of relationships to a fulfilling life. But there is a limit to what it can do. Money is a problem. There is not enough playing-field space. Science laboratories are cramped and ill-equipped. Classes are too large. Good teachers are not always easy to recruit.

At the other end of the city, children at Minority School have all the facilities they need – a good library, an indoor swimming pool, large grounds, personal tuition, time and opportunities to develop their own interests . . . Happily, most alumni from both schools do reasonably well in later life, according to the criteria of well-being presented in this book.

Those from Majority tend to find more fulfilment in their relationships – their family lives and friendships – than in their work. They have little time to explore the cultural worlds their school opened up for them, and in time their taste for these tends to dissolve away. Most of them are not well off. The basics of life – getting work, doing chores, food and heating bills, living space, coping with health problems – are a source of anxiety and take up a lot of their time. Even so, compared with people much worse off elsewhere in the world, even with their own grandparents, they live well.

Minority's graduates live even better. Most of them are in well-paid jobs they enjoy. They spend less time on basic needs and more on intrinsic goods. Relationships figure prominently among these, but they have a host of other interests, too, some of them costly. Even with the more free time they tend to have compared with Majority people, there is never enough to throw themselves into all life's pleasures.

The point of this parable is not social critique – although it may ring a few bells – but the more theoretical consideration that it would not be *enough* to make well-being aims pivotal to a school's activity. Even if they were, and everyone enjoyed a minimum level of well-being as a result, some could still far outsoar this and get much more out of life than others.

For some social planners this would not be a problem. The key thing for them is that there be a safety net below which no one can fall. Above this, they'll tell you, there are bound to be differences: only an ideologically driven egalitarian would seek to iron them all out.

I have some sympathy with their distaste for this kind of egalitarianism. But only to a point. Should the fact that men in Blackpool tend to live ten years less than those in Chelsea trouble us? Our anti-egalitarian may say 'So what? 73 years is surely a good-enough innings'. What makes the softer-hearted, *Guardian*-reading citizen want to do more is her thought that ten years is a large proportion of a human life, and it is distressing that those already well placed to put their time allotment to good use are so advantaged. One month's discrepancy may not trouble her, but *ten years*?

In education policy, we should try to ensure that our rallying cry of 'well-being for all' does *not* allow gross discrepancies like this.

Schools and families

As soon as she is born, Willow is enveloped in close, loving relationships. In the course of her first year or so, as she becomes capable of intentional action, her parents initiate her into activities like playing peek-a-boo, pushing small cars down curly plastic chutes and turning over the pages of touchy-scratchy books. They are delighted by the gusto with which she hurls herself into these pursuits and by her rapidly increasing proficiency in them.

If a flourishing life is one spent in whole-hearted and successful engagement in worthwhile relationships and activities, toddler Willow is already some way down the road. Although she seems in a world of her own as she pushes her toddle truck around the garden, she also loves helping to feed the ducks by the lake at Ally Pally, joining in pillow and duvet romps and putting her wooden bricks back in the toy box when asked to do so. Co-operative activities like these are teaching her, although she is only on the edge of understanding it, that her own well-being and that of others are closely intertwined. When, sitting in her highchair, she throws her slice of pizza onto the kitchen floor, she looks at the unhappy face of her grandma and her own expression grows sad too. Again, she is learning, without yet properly knowing it, that whether things are going well or ill for those close to her *matters* to her.

As Willow grows older, her parents and carers lay further foundations for her well-being. They do simple jigsaws with her, play ball with her in the park, read stories to her and show her the pigs and goats at Wimpole Hall Farm. She is extending the range of her activities and deepening her engagement in them.

She is, as yet, far from a full-blown autonomous person. She is not able to make informed worthwhile choices and resolve conflicts between alternatives. Yet she is given plenty of freedom in deciding what to do and, as she learns to speak, is encouraged to talk about her likes and dislikes.

She is also far from being a full-blown democratic citizen. Yet, even as a young child, she is being acculturated into a world of reason-giving and treating others with respect, which are the first steps towards this.

Parents and carers help her to make sense of the world around her. They encourage her delight at frogs, furry caterpillars and other joys of the natural world. They play imaginative games with her, develop her nascent sense of humour. And all the time they are shaping the kind of person she is, getting her to be self-confident, self-reliant, patient and helpful to other people. They let her know that she cannot always get her way, keep her from too much inappropriate food or drink and do not make a fuss over little knocks and falls.

In all these ways, by immersion in activities and relationships, by developing her understanding of the world, imagination and a range of personal dispositions, they are, bit by bit, providing her with much of what she will need to have a fulfilling life.

School, on this model, is a natural extension of such a home. It is governed by the same overarching aim, to help children to live abundantly and help others to do so. Learning to read opens up for them new landscapes of worthwhile activity, feeding both the imagination and the understanding. They learn to operate with numbers, explore all kinds of new practical activities and find out more about the work that people do, are inducted as proto-citizens into collective discussion of important matters.

Because they are following the same overall aim, teachers and parents, like those in the fable, work closely together. They each have a hand in every major aspect of upbringing – in making sure the child is enthusiastically and successfully engaged in activities and relationships; in extending these for her in range and depth; in encouraging her, as she grows more capable of this, to make autonomous choices about what she engages in; in furthering her understanding of the social and natural worlds around her; in bringing her to see her well-being as intimately connected with that of other people; and in developing the personal qualities necessary to her well-being as an individual and as a citizen in the making.

There are differences between parents and teachers too, of course. Teachers do not know the child as intimately as the parent. Parents do not have the time or the knowledge that teachers collectively have to extend the child's experience in numerous directions. But it would be wrong to exaggerate the differences and minimise overlaps. The work of both groups is guided by the same general aims. The more collaboration between them, the more seamless and harmonious the child's education is likely to become.

We would also do well to narrow the gap, where it exists, between teachers and parents. Dramatically reducing class sizes is a priority. Classes of 30 might make sense in a regime devoted to simple skill acquisition or rote learning, but the more personal the education becomes, the more you need smaller groups. Good fee-paying schools and the parents who pay them know this well. That is why they go for classes of 15, not twice that number. Until the present recession, Scottish state education was heading fast in the same direction, following calls for classes of 18 in the first three primary years.

On the other side of the argument, some research has shown little apparent improvement in performance between class sizes of 18–25. This may be music to the ears of those who don't want to spend more on state education. But it is within the system as we know it. And this has been driven by other values than the well-being I have been defending in this book. Jan

Comenius, a seventeenth-century founding father of the traditional academic curriculum, was all for efficiency. Once you follow his method of teaching, everything is possible. 'I maintain,' he said, 'that it is not only possible for one teacher to teach several hundred scholars at once, but that it is also essential; since for both the teachers and their pupils it is by far the most advantageous system' (Comenius, 1638/1907: 164). Not even the most cheese-paring tax-reducer will go as far as this today, but the paraphernalia of efficiency – pupils sitting quietly in desks listening to teachers, the 'one sure method' of teaching reading, the testing, the incitements to compete – are hardly without their advocates.

If education is just knowledge transmission, the scope for mechanising it is at its greatest. Geometry is no respecter of individuality. The circumference of a circle is $2\pi r$ for the sexually obsessed 13-year-old as for the child still into shell collecting. The more impersonal the system, the more we can go along with Comenius. The more our sights are on well-being, the more unanswerable the case for smaller classes.

Taking aims seriously

What curriculum best suits the schools we have in mind? It is likely to diverge from the traditional subject-based one. I looked at this briefly in Part 1, Chapter 2, in the shape of the English National Curriculum. There I noted the weight put on the acquisition of scientific, mathematical, historical, and geographical knowledge, with less on the arts and personal and civic life. Later chapters reinforced the oddness of this ordering.

We need to rethink the curriculum. Its weakness is that those who defend it begin in the wrong place – with a list of subjects. The *right* place to begin is with overall aims. In education, as in any other practical enterprise, from making furniture to medicine, you have to begin with some idea of where you are going. You don't start with means to ends – gluing pieces of wood together or using a stethoscope. You take off from basic purposes – making something to sit on, promoting health. In education, it's the same. You don't start with *structures* within which learning can take place – modern foreign languages or music as timetabled subjects – but with what schools are *for*.

Once you have decided to make something to sit on, the next step is to design something suitable. What material will you use? You go for wood, rather than metal or plastic. What sort of wood? What will the end-product look like? How will the pieces be shaped and fixed together?

It is the same for education. It's more complicated, because specifying the aim is much harder. Suppose we agree that this should mainly be about equipping children to lead a fulfilling life. What it *is* to lead such a life is not easy to spell out. It has, after all, taken me the best part of the book to hack a rough path through the forest.

The next step is to design something to fit this bill. What kinds of learning are most suitable? What personal qualities do we want in children? What do they need to understand? What mental and physical skills should they have?

I say more below about how this abstract schema might be filled in. But one thing should be obvious already: the upshot of the complex and delicate enquiry this requires is unlikely to be a curriculum carved neatly into the familiar subjects.

This makes no sense. Learning neat, within a school subject, is *one* way of learning, but not the only one. Practical projects, discussion, everyday experience, habituation . . . there are countless forms that learning can take. Why privilege the traditional?

I've combed through everything I know to find some valid reason for a subject-structured curriculum, but so far I have drawn a blank. You can try to *explain* why its hold on our thinking has become so powerful, but a solid *justification* is a different matter. I won't go into either of these areas now, since I have discussed both at length in *The Invention of the Secondary Curriculum* (White, forthcoming).

In case, like the *Daily Mail* on one occasion, you get me wrong, I'm not at all arguing that children should learn *no* history, science, geography or mathematics. On the contrary, they will need induction into all of these if they are to live a full life. My only gripe is with a system that makes these categories sacrosanct, that starts and finishes its curricular planning with a structure of discrete subjects.

Let me illustrate. History is a subject whose teaching in British secondary schools has changed over the last 50 years, and changed for the better. Half a century ago, it was inward-looking, transmitting facts, largely about British political history, to largely passive students (Husbands *et al.*, 2003). These days there is more active learning, more socially relevant content, more attentiveness to wider educational purposes (10–12). Teachers of the subject overwhelmingly see it now as promoting moral and civic ends rather than as something to be studied for its own sake. They are concerned with 'the teaching of values such as toleration, respect for diversity, understanding of different attitudes and beliefs' (123).

This is an undoubted advance. Whether teachers of mathematics, science and foreign languages are so attuned to wider social purposes is another matter, but at least the historians have shown that change is possible.

But there are rocks ahead for the subject specialist. For if moral and civic ends are where you start, and not internal departure platforms within history itself, then what priority should historical studies of the slave trade or Islam have among the countless other, *non-historical*, ways in which respect for diversity and other virtues may be promoted? Once subject specialists leave their boxes and are into larger purposes, they put at risk the sacrosanct position of their own discipline within the curriculum.

The British school curriculum is out of joint. Its subjects, with a few additions unloved by traditionalists, are the same as those prescribed for the secondary school since the 1860s. The twentieth century has seen their empire spread beyond a tiny fraction of the population to encompass, since 1988, not only all secondary pupils but also most primary children as well. Concomitantly, they have each become a fortress within the curriculum, timetable-walled against invaders, strong in their professional bonds within subject associations and reinforced by their role within the examination structure.

This is why recent reforms of the curriculum have done little to erode their might. The impressive set of overall aims attached to the National Curriculum in 1999 had no discernible impact on content within the subjects. A second shot at an aims-based curriculum, in 2007, was half-hearted at best, and in any case hamstrung by government's insistence that the subjects stay untouched. If an aims-based approach is to be taken seriously, vehicles by which aims are to be realised should not be prejudged. School subjects, it bears repeating, are only one kind among many.

It has been no surprise to the educational world that the ministers of education within the post-May 2010 Coalition, Michael Gove and Nick Gibb, have come out so emphatically in favour of school subjects and, in the case of history, of traditional priorities within them. What motivates these conservatives may be no more than, well, conservatism, in the sense of attachment to what has happened in the past. But there may be more to it. When I was a child, after the end of the Second World War, the curriculum in question had been, for decades, closely associated with the grammar school and the 10–20 per cent of children, mainly from the middle classes, that went to it. Those educated in this way tended to pass on to their children the attitudes they needed to succeed within this system, notably diligence in mastering whatever they were expected to learn, without dreaming of asking what it was all for.

Now that this curriculum is mandatory for all, this (now much larger) group of people has the edge over families lacking this history of involvement in academic learning. This fact is widely recognised, even in right-wing circles. The right-of-centre think-tank Civitas, for instance, states, in a recent publication on the National Curriculum (Conway, 2010: 71):

> It may well be true that, in general, the more socially privileged the background from which children come the easier they find it to master a traditional curriculum. Hence it may well be that children from more privileged backgrounds tend to fare better on assessment on such a curriculum than children from less privileged backgrounds.

It would not be at all surprising, then, if politicians allied to the more privileged groups resisted reformers' attempts to put the curriculum on a different footing.

We come back to a central theme of this book. It is possible, in an affluent country like Britain, to arrange things so that everyone, not just a favoured section of the population, is equipped, through education and other means, to lead a full, rich life. Attachment to old curriculum patterns is an obstacle to this.

One of my favourite Monty Python sketches showed a group of Welsh coalminers working deep underground and heatedly discussing different interpretations of the Hundred Years War. I thought of this again on my walk to the newsagents and back this morning. I passed a gardener, a window cleaner, a taxi driver, men putting in a loft room, workmen from Barnet Council Parks Department, several small shop owners. How valuable to all these, assuming they experienced it, was their traditional academic curriculum? How much benefit did they derive from their French lessons, their geometry, their history of the Middle Ages?

Don't, please, take the sceptical attitude you rightly pick out in these remarks as a sign that I think ordinary people's education should be trimmed back to next-to-nothing. On the contrary, I'd like to see schools providing *for everyone* an education far richer and more challenging than most have now. This makes good sense if, as a community, we want everyone to have the wherewithal for a fulfilling life, including adequate income and free time, and easy access to post-school adult education at all levels.

In moving to something closer to the mark, we need to base education on an appropriate set of aims. When I say 'base', I mean this literally. I am *not* saying 'The traditional subjects aren't enough; they need to be accompanied by an overall aims statement'. We have had such aims statements for the last ten years and they have made precious little difference. That is because the subjects are still as entrenched as they ever were. 'Basing' school education on overall aims means *following through* from the initial, more general, aims to more and more determinate sub-aims. Some of these are likely to lead us towards material currently included in school subjects; others elsewhere. I will be saying more in the next two sections about how this might shape up.

Well-being aims: a first look

If home and school education is to equip everyone to lead a flourishing life, what, more precisely, is it to do? Summarising discussions in Part 1, we can say something like the following.

Education for well-being involves preparing children for a life of autonomous, whole-hearted and successful engagement in worthwhile activities and relationships (Chapter 8). Parents and teachers will want them to make their own choices about these (p. 64). This means acquainting them, partly drawing on their powers of imagination, with an array of future possible options. But it also means children engaging *now* in worthwhile pursuits.

This generates a tension between breadth and engagement. There is a case for putting more weight on the latter (see Chapters 7, p. 55; 8, p. 64).

Being an *autonomous* agent involves much more than the two-year-old's ability to choose between playing with his diggers or his train set. It requires personal qualities and levels of understanding still far beyond him (Chapter 8, p. 61). I say more about these below. At the same time, his kind of choosing is the starting point for more considered and informed choices later.

If *whole-heartedness* is key to well-being (Chapter 8, p. 60), we should expect to find it permeating every learning activity. It is not enough for children to grind in a dutiful way through tasks set for them, however impressive their achievements. Whole-hearted enjoyment will be a more valued aim than it often is in schools today (Chapters 6, p. 47; 7, p. 55; 8, p. 64). There should be less boredom, switching off, divided attention and classroom disruption – especially among pupils for whom the academic grind has no light at the end of its tunnel. In this as in other things, school life would become closer to the good family life sketched in Chapter 15 above.

Success – in the shape of successful engagement – is an educational and social ideal applicable to everybody: barring ill-luck and misjudgement, everyone's life should be a success, not a failure (Chapter 6, p. 45). This has nothing to do with fame or celebrity (Chapter 5), or with ending up with higher-than-average income and social status (Chapter 8, p. 59). It does not require following a life plan (Chapter 9, p. 75).

Both parents and teachers need to be clear on what count as intrinsically *worthwhile* pursuits. They have to avoid two extremes. First, that any activity is as valuable as any other provided it is in line with one's informed preferences (Chapter 7); second, that only activities within a restricted range are *really* worthwhile – certain intellectual or cultural activities, for instance (Chapter 8, p. 66). There is a strong case for keeping the range much wider. It includes work activities of all kinds, paid and unpaid, provided that other conditions, of autonomy and whole-heartedness, are met (Chapter 9). It embraces co-operative and other activities intended to further other people's well-being, either face-to-face or at the civic level (Chapter 10). Personal relationships, especially those of friendship and intimacy, are also vital elements in flourishing, and schools and families should do what they can to equip children for these (Chapter 8, p. 67).

Teachers and parents need to have well-grounded confidence in their judgements about worthwhileness and to pass this on to their children/pupils. There is a direct link here with the strengthening of a democratic society, given that this kind of polity requires ongoing discussion, on as wide a front as possible, and among those inside the issues, of what makes a human life worth living (Chapter 11). Among other things, parents and teachers will be acquainting young people with deeper as well as surface levels of enjoyment and involvement, making sure that learners keep in touch with the world of common human concerns and not lose themselves in too blinkered a way within some technical specialism (Chapter 12).

The arts, especially literature, are significant here (Chapter 12, p. 105). There is a case for giving them a higher profile. The curricular tradition in which we have been brought up has especially prized the acquisition of knowledge and insufficiently valued aesthetic and imaginative pursuits. Even today, artistic subjects, not least literature, are to some extent assimilated to the 'knowledge' tradition. Our system of testing and examining rewards the ability to critically assess a text rather than enjoyable immersion in it. Until recently, all 14-year-olds in English maintained schools had to sit national tests on a play by Shakespeare, like *Macbeth*, and answer factual questions on plot and characterisation.

In an age when religious notions of fulfilment carry less weight, and we see the life we have as its only stage (Chapters 2, 3, 13), it is not surprising that the arts – as well as natural beauty – should mean so much to us. It is easy, given appropriate direction, to become captivated by the worlds of sensuous delight and human interest that painters, musicians, poets and other artists create for us, and into which they deliberately seduce us. It is easier for most of us to get absorbed in the arts in this way than it is to develop a like passion for mathematics or chemistry. Part of the artistry of art, notably, again, literature, is the passage it forges for us, from the sounds and other sensuous objects it brings before us – in actuality or via the imagination – to deeper levels of feeling and reflection.

The primacy of dispositions

Education for well-being is built around acquiring personal qualities (dispositions) on the one hand and understanding on the other. The two go together. As understanding deepens and becomes more extensive, a child's dispositions are enriched. Of the two, dispositions are more important. For parents and teachers, the first consideration is the kind of person a child is becoming. They will want her to be, among other things, helpful, enjoyably involved in what she is doing, able to cope with adversity, humorous, imaginative, confident, wary – where appropriate – of other people.

I say something rather more systematic in a moment about acquiring qualities like these. What should most exercise us initially is not that the child becomes proficient in French, or knows about the atomic structure of matter, or be able to solve algebraic equations. These things may or may not be important in her education, but if they are, they come into view at a different place. The starting point is that she should have the positive qualities needed for a flourishing life. We would not want her to become brilliant at algebra and Latin, but also cripplingly anxious, or cynical, or a sadist. First things first.

It would also be wrong to take the line that only parents do person-making, and only teachers academic learning. Both parties are educators; and both should be working to the same goals. The foremost of these are to do with personal qualities.

I discussed in Part 1 Chapter 4 various necessary conditions of a flourishing life like shelter, good health, a minimum income and freedom. In certain of these areas, parents and teachers need to build up desirable dispositions.

Take health. Human beings are biological organisms, not just minds. Here, as elsewhere, schools have some catching up to do. They have been used to dealing only with children's mental powers in a narrow sense of this term – with their assimilating information, linking ideas, systematising, deducing, summarising, remembering. In doing so, they have traditionally paid next-to-no attention to their physicality, tethering it in desks so as to interfere as little as possible with the work of the intellect.

Like Aristotle, the great pre-Christian thinker whose understanding of human nature was rooted in biology, in getting clear about our well-being we should begin with our innate bodily desires and emotions, and the habituation we all need in managing them well. In recent years, schools have moved a little in this direction in the work they do on health education and emotional learning. The pity is that this is often merely tacked on to what some see as the 'real' curriculum, sometimes as an emergency reaction to a perceived social crisis among the young – drug-taking, teenage pregnancy, obesity, antisocial behaviour.

We need to step back. We are all born with bodily desires – for food, drink, elimination, physical activity, sex, rest – that we have to learn to manage. This starts in infancy through parental training and continues throughout childhood and adolescence, with young people themselves taking increasingly autonomous control. This involves their learning to make sensible judgements, not easily encompassed by simple rules, about what to do, how and when.

For a fuller account of how this works, using eating as an example, see Part 1 Chapter 4. We saw there how this kind of behavioural learning progressively benefits from the greater understanding that children come to have of the nature of different foodstuffs and their benefits for and risks to health; of social appropriateness; of the need to be flexible according to circumstance; of social and commercial pressures on them to eat inappropriately. Parallel points can be made about other physical desires. There is every reason to group these desires together in our educational thinking – and *no* reason to keep PE, school dinners and sex education hived off from each other in their current separate boxes.

A similar pattern – early habituation, increasing understanding and intelligent judgment, reaction and action according to circumstances – also applies to the management of innate emotions like fear, anger and joy, as well as to more culturally dependent emotions like resentment, shame, anxiety, feelings of high or low self-esteem, trust, confidence, warmth and love towards others. As with their physical desires, children will make all sorts of mistakes along the way. The process is not the simplistic one, traditionally favoured, of keeping firm clamps on one's feelings. It is far more subtle and delicate – coming to understand in relation to anger, for example, on what occasions it is appropriate to feel it or display it or act on it; to what degree; to whom; and in what ways. I do not need to underline the role that literature can play, via the imagination, in this refinement of our emotions. This reinforces my message above about making the arts more prominent in education.

Managing our emotions can be important for our health. Think of a severe anxiety or depression associated with low self-esteem. But it is essential beyond this, in making the most of the activities and relationships that fill our lives. Education for well-being is in large part the shaping of *love* – love of our work, of nature, gardening, reading fiction, cycling, or whatever other activities grab us, and the manifold types of love we learn to feel towards other people at different levels of intimacy or non-intimacy. These person-directed kinds of love are closely connected with other virtues that parents and teachers should be encouraging: respect for others' autonomy, recognition, mutual aid, honesty, fairness, friendliness, kindness, good humour, civic concern.

Whatever we love, and however we shape our unique path through life as an autonomous agent, we all have to acquire dispositions of a more general kind, whose function is to keep our lives focused appropriately, and held together in some sort of unity.

On the topic of focus, in carrying out many kinds of project we need persistence, confidence, flexibility in reacting to different circumstances, and the ability to cope with obstacles and overcome them.

On the topic of unity, given the multitude of different values we come to acquire, all of which have some call on us, we have to have some way of judging their relative importance to us at different points. This takes us away from whatever it is we are actively engaged in and into reflection. Sometimes this is over more trivial matters – How am I going to spend the free evening ahead? – and sometimes at a deeper or more conflict-ridden level – Am I getting too attached to my work at the expense of my friends?

There are balances to be struck, too, between the amount of time I put into reflectiveness as against single-hearted involvement in relationships and activities themselves. As with any disposition, we have to avoid the inappropriate – on the one hand, getting so caught up in our pursuits that we do not stop to think things over when thinking is necessary; and on the other, losing ourselves in over-reflectiveness.

As children's value worlds with all their conflicts grow richer, they need to rely more and more on this reflective virtue. How are they to acquire it? Having eschewed the personal for the academic, traditional education leaves it in the shadows. But there is every reason why today's teachers and parents should bring it into the light.

The same goes for other, overlapping, unity-related virtues. A sense of perspective, for instance. For each of us, our values come to form something like a hierarchy, although not usually a very systematic one. I like eating choc-ices, playing with my grandson, writing about education, watching TV detective series, going to philosophy seminars, hearing gossip, drinking Cinzano, reading poetry, and countless other things. I try to keep things in proportion, spending more time on what, for me, are the more important things, trying to avoid temptations to eat too much, watch too much TV, allow myself to get overwhelmed by some perceived slight, or get too involved in the newspaper when I should be getting on with my writing. As their value-worlds become richer, young people, like all of us, need to learn perspective. Again, this should not be left to chance.

Those who see schools as purveying-grounds of knowledge rarely champion one of its most important branches – self-knowledge. It is not difficult, like Emma in Jane Austen's novel, to become a victim of self-deception. As with a sense of perspective, being with other people who can help us to see what we are really like – our own Mr Knightleys – is a well-trodden path to self-awareness. This is the master-virtue that keeps us in touch with what most matters to us. It should not be confused with self-absorption; and the point made earlier about excessive reflectiveness is also apposite here.

As we saw in Chapter 12, self-knowledge is, above all, a practical virtue, concerned with our overall self-guidance through life. It is more important to us than the knowledge of volcanoes or the future tense of French verbs prized within the academic educational tradition. As such, it is central to the well-being school. It thrives on everyday intercourse with others, literature and film, discussion and opportunities for private reflection and self-expression.

Knowledge and understanding

Apart from self-knowledge, understanding our social and natural worlds is a large part of anyone's education. But should we structure it as we do? We standardly cut areas of knowledge up into discipline-sized blocks – mathematics, history, the sciences etc. The internal organisation of each subject block is left to its experts. These each have their own cleavers, dividing elementary mathematics, say, into arithmetic, algebra and geometry, and making further sub-classifications within these. Recently, as we saw with history, there have been moves to make subjects more responsive to outside aims, but older patterns persist. 'Britain 1066–1500' is still a ubiquitous module for the first year of secondary school.

An alternative way of selecting knowledge begins from general aims. Take, as an example, the disposition described above as 'a sense of perspective'. One reason why children sometimes find this hard to acquire is pressure on them from peer groups and the media to make certain desires – for celebrity, alcohol, fatty foods, sex, fashion goods – crowd out others. They need to *understand* these pressures, and the financial interests behind them.

Wherever we start among general aims, knowledge and understanding soon come into the picture. Work on health-related basic needs depends on knowledge about our biological make-up; relationships education, on insight into how people think and feel. Learners need some understanding of the world of employment, including its career options, as part of a wider array of possible worthwhile activities.

These are only one or two examples. The last reminds us that one of the things young people will need is some understanding of the society in which they live. This includes not only the world of work and the economy, but also welfare services, political arrangements and differences of lifestyle and opportunities based on class, region, religion and ethnic background. Some of these knowledge requirements take us into familiar school subjects like history and geography, as well as the mathematics and science needed to get inside social statistics and the technological bases of the economy. But:

(a) as subject content is determined via overall aims, it may well differ from conventional practice. For 12-year-olds studying history, 'Britain 1066–1500' may be less fit for purpose than projects on, say, changes over the last century in the transport infrastructure, or immigrant communities, or the position of women in society;

(b) a lot of the knowledge children need comes from elsewhere than the usual subjects. Children need to know something about the media, about money management, the political system, their own and others' nature, shrinking world resources, the structure of employment, class and ethnic divisions, the ethical and aesthetic values associated with well-being.

We have to be careful. There is no end to the knowledge that *could* be beneficial to children and that they *could* acquire at school. I am not denying for a moment that much of their school life will be dedicated to knowledge acquisition. But this must be subordinate to aims mentioned earlier in this chapter, not least whole-heartedness of engagement in valuable pursuits.

Rethinking the curriculum

All this speaks for radical changes in curriculum planning. In England, as often elsewhere, there is a national curriculum built largely around traditional subjects. Thinking about wider aims is pushed to the margins or welded awkwardly onto an existing structure.

But this gets things the wrong way round. School subjects are not ends in themselves, but vehicles – and not the only ones – to attain further purposes.

The role of the state is not to prescribe vehicles, but to provide an overall picture of what education should be about. How overall aims are best realised is something best left to professionals – to teachers who intelligently work out what kind of learning structures are best for children of *these* kinds, living in *this* kind of community and facing *these* kinds of obstacles and opportunities. Despite their predilection for interfering in the details of what subject content should be taught, politicians lack the on-the-ground knowledge to make such judgements.

Where the political sphere *does* come into play is in indicating what education should be for. This is essentially a political issue since it is intimately connected with the kind of society we wish to bring about or maintain. In a democracy of equal citizens, teachers have no special, privileged voice on this. Postmen, housewives, shopkeepers and pensioners have the same stake as any teacher.

The state should determine the larger aims; schools, the means of realising them. But what, here, is 'the state'? The government in power? If so, what is to stop ministers imposing their idiosyncratic preferences? There is a case for some kind of regularly convened national commission, at arm's length from politicians' pressure, that works out, in no haste, what the aims should be. Its guiding principle should be appropriateness for a liberal-democratic society. In this, a central value is the well-being of each citizen.

The commission would not produce its conclusions out of the blue. A large part of its remit would be wide consultation and the promotion of public debate. Also fitting its democratic context would be an onus on it not to come up with a mere *list* of aims, but to back up any recommendations with a full and considered rationale. Over time, new sets of aims would replace the old as existing rationales were subjected to public critique.

Chapter 17

Education for well-being: learning arrangements

I turn now from ends to means, from overall aims to ways schools adopt to realise them.

Well-being as a school subject

In Part I Chapter 1, I mentioned ways in which English secondary schools have begun promoting pupils' well-being through lessons and programmes specifically devoted to it. A well-known example is Wellington College's course of lessons on well-being (or 'happiness'). Less headline-hitting has been the arrival of a new statutory subject called *Personal wellbeing*. This is twinned with *Economic wellbeing and financial capability*.

I refrain from critical assessment of specifics. This is partly because others are already doing this (Suissa, 2008). It is also partly because, for the most part, I have no quarrel with the programmes I have seen. *Personal wellbeing*, for instance, includes work on confidence, healthy lifestyles, relationships, risk and social diversity that chimes with many of the themes in this book.

My main worry is at another level. The issue is *not* that there is an area – to do with personal fulfilment – that has not been covered by traditional subjects and now deserves a subject slot of its own. To think this way is to think in the old way. It assumes we have to start from subjects. If we began with fundamental purposes – that is, if the curriculum were aims-based rather than subject-based – we should soon see that everything, or nearly everything, that a school does should help to equip children for a fulfilling life. Making personal well-being a separate subject may not be helpful. It may confirm more traditional teachers of other subjects in their belief that their first duty is to their own discipline. In addition, as no one subject can hope to respond to all the manifold aspects of well-being that this book has revealed, the content of the separate subject in question is likely to be very selective. This is true of the new National Curriculum subject *Personal wellbeing*. It deals especially with confidence, health, relationships, risk and diversity. These are important; but concentrating its efforts on these leaves so much more untouched.

The place of subjects

I have little to add on this. Schools should be given maximum freedom to decide how best to realise overall aims, including well-being aims. They should be free to organise their work within discrete subjects, via interdisciplinary or other kinds of projects, or in other ways, not least whole-school processes. English schools have, *in fact*, been free in this way since the National Curriculum appeared in 1988. They have had to conform to statutory requirements arranged subject by subject; but how they meet these, whether by keeping within subjects or not, has been up to them. Despite this latitude, secondary schools more than primaries have generally worked within a subject framework. This is not surprising, given that secondary teachers are trained in teaching particular subjects and employed within subject departments in schools. We should now look for ways to encourage schools to think outside these boxes.

Compulsion and choice

As things are, children normally *have* to engage, at times not of their choosing, in prescribed curricular activities. Sometimes they find these absorbing. But very often they do not. They may not be interested in doing French just at the times set for this, although they may enjoy it in other circumstances. Or they find it hard to get on with French, whatever the circumstances, even though they willingly get caught up in drama or music.

The more time pupils spend at school doing things they don't have their heart in, the more counter-productive this is from a well-being point of view. One way of making things better would be to improve the quality of teaching and teacher training so that teachers know better how to motivate children to love their subject. Another would be to teach compulsory lessons in appealing ways, for instance through themes and projects as well as subjects. A third would be still to insist on comprehensive coverage but leave children freer to choose what they do and when. A fourth would be not to let comprehensiveness win out over whole-hearted engagement (see p. 129, 'Well-being aims: a first look'), but to give children from an early age expanding opportunities to choose what they want to explore further.

Some combination of all these may be the way to go. Giving children more freedom to organise their work is especially important. The internet can be a resource here. Professor Sugata Mitra of Newcastle University works with primary children using computers in self-organised groups of four or five to answer a question designed by a teacher, and left free to work, or not, as they please. Mitra asked ten-year-olds from Turin, for instance, 'Who was Pythagoras, and what did he do?' Twenty minutes later, he tells us, 'every group had right-angled triangles up on screen. One group was beginning to examine the equation of squares.' In another school, in

Gateshead, ten-year-olds working to the same self-organising model were given GCSE questions, normally studied by pupils five years older – and usually got the answer right (*Education Guardian*, 19 October 2010).

There is no case for the libertarian project of allowing children maximum choice (see Part 1, Chapter 7). But there is everything to be said for building in more free time for children to do their own thing, including, if they wish, occasionally mooning around and daydreaming.

Working and learning

Is school a place for work or for learning (see Chapter 9)? These often go together: children acquire knowledge, hone skills, become more entrenched in habits in the course of producing solutions to problems, essays, paintings. But sometimes they generate end-products but learn nothing in the process: reception pupils can be sitting around their table cutting out yet more identical paper dolls; older students filling in worksheets when already familiar with the material. Not all learning comes via work. Think of what we can all pick up from everyday experience, from reading for enjoyment, from watching films and from conversation. If schools are places for whole-hearted engagement in activities, sometimes these will involve work, sometimes not.

This requires a shift from the traditional view of schools as workplaces, where children engage in carefully structured activities – doing sums, listening to the teacher, committing things to memory, writing – with certain end-products in mind. School work, homework and exam preparation together habituate them to a regime of largely heteronomous work. Although when young children first come to school they spend a lot of time playing, within a couple of years they are brought to see that school is a more serious business.

The origins of this notion of schooling go back to Protestant educational ideas and practices of the seventeenth century, found in Comenius and others. It went with the high value placed on obligatory work as a sign of one's suitability for salvation. Echoes of this occur today in the common idea that schools should prepare young people for the 'harsh realities' of adult life.

Some pupils put up with the rigours of school life not because they like the idea of a life of heteronomous work but because they see hard heteronomous work today as a passport to autonomous work tomorrow – as a doctor, an academic, an architect, a writer. For them, school work may indeed help to equip them – in an instrumental way – for a life of autonomous well-being.

Many other pupils lack the family support to help them over the hurdles. They get discouraged, see themselves as failures. From the point of view of preparation for a fulfilling life, their schooling is counter-productive.

There is a strong case for making it more fit for purpose. Whole-heartedness of involvement is the watchword. Sometimes this is in non-work activities; sometimes it is end-product-directed. Work as experienced against the grain rather than as something one really wants to do is kept to a minimum. As far as possible, school work is autonomous – something learners freely choose to do.

Collaborative and solitary learning

Traditionally, schools have been places where children work as individuals. Hence the customary arrangement of fixed classroom furniture, with pupils sitting in rows or separate desks under the teacher's eye. Today, more flexible arrangements are commonplace, with movable tables suiting both individual and group work. This is in line with the non-atomic nature of personal well-being as described in Chapter 10. If one's own flourishing is intimately tied in with other people's, this gives schools an excellent intrinsic reason for encouraging collaborative learning for shared ends. Sugata Mitra's work, described above, is an example.

This is not to demean solitary learning. This can take different forms. Conventionally, the learner is in a classroom full of other students. She is far from alone, far from being able to take her thoughts and feelings where she will. She is part of a collection of individuals, all of whom have to keep to the programme their teacher has arranged for them. She is aware of the presence of her classmates, sometimes in a background way, sometimes focally, as friends, rivals or clowns.

Her experience will not be absent from the well-being school. Some learning will lend itself to it. But there will be much more room for a different kind of solitary learning. Think of how we learn as adults. In my own school days, I was introduced to Shakespeare in classes surrounded by other boys. Two legacies from those days: a few remembered lines like 'Old John of Gaunt, time-honoured Lancaster', and little desire to take things further. Recently, having time on my hands, I decided to read all Shakespeare's works in chronological order. Now into *Julius Caesar*, I am finding the experience extraordinarily absorbing. I have a self-chosen programme; I start and stop as I will, let my thoughts take off, interweave my reading with visits to the theatre, rejoice in freedom of spirit. I am sure we can do more to prevent school students so often having to work in lock-step by creating room for this kind of solitary freedom.

This is not at odds with what I was saying about collaborative learning. This can sometimes be as hidebound as the way I learnt *Richard II*. Within obvious limits, the more freedom children have to shape the way their shared project on local care for the elderly is going, the more spaces they have in which they can let their imagination, feelings and reasoning powers take wing, the better.

Discussion

One form of collaborative learning is discussion. Earlier in the book, I have shown how it can help pupils, as part of their education in citizenship, towards a clearer perspective on what their own and other people's well-being consists in. There is so much confusion within the culture about this that, unless educators take steps to separate the strands and focus attention on the soundness of arguments, many youngsters will leave school with misleading or jumbled views.

Topics picked out in Part 1 as suitable for class discussion include the following. Where is one's well-being located, in this world or another? More basic considerations on which this rests: the possibility of an afterlife; the existence of God (Chapter 2); meeting basic needs as a prerequisite of one's flourishing; meeting people's basic needs more generally, at national and global levels (Chapter 3). What place do fame and wealth have in human flourishing? What counts as a successful life? (Chapter 5). Is it the life of pleasure? What light can the story of the 'experience machine' cast on this? (Chapter 6). Are we as individuals in the best position to know what makes for the fulfilling life? (Chapter 7). How important is whole-hearted involvement in activities and relationships? How might schools have to change to accommodate this? (Chapter 8). What place does work have in a fulfilling life? (Chapter 9). If I am to flourish, must I always be looking out for Number One? Are my own well-being and moral demands on me necessarily in conflict? (Chapter 10). Is there an objective foundation for well-being? Are there people we can turn to as reliable authorities on how we should live? What messages is our own school sending through to us about this? (Chapter 11). Do some worthwhile activities have greater depth than others? What counts as depth? Do the arts and humanities have a special place? (Chapter 12). Does human life have a meaning? What light does evolution theory throw on this? Can life be meaningful if it has no external purpose? (Chapter 13).

Some of these topics may be suitable only for older learners. But even with very young ones we can make a start. Values-orientated work in the area of philosophy for children often revolves around discussions of things like fame, wealth, friendship and happiness. In his recent book on secondary education, *How to Teach*, Phil Beadle (2010: 103–44) entertainingly and usefully describes ways of organising discussions and pitfalls to avoid.

Assessment

How is education for well-being to be assessed? School assessment as we know it is yoked to our knowledge-centred tradition. It demands evidence of how much and how well pupils have learnt, mainly through written work – as homework or as performance in in-school tests and public examinations. Its distant origins are in religion – in giving an account to God via his representatives of how far one has progressed spiritually in countering the sin of ignorance. Today, assessment has different purposes: diagnosis, to see how best to help learners overcome obstacles and move on; accountability, to judge how schools are doing, with public expenditure and parental choice in mind; post-school objectives – to help students compete for jobs or university and college places.

How conducive is our present system to the pupil's well-being? Diagnostic assessment is clearly a good thing, assuming that what is assessed is valuable from a well-being point of view. Whether it is or not depends on issues raised earlier, especially about the space given to knowledge in education. But summative forms of assessment, like SATs, GCSE or A-level exams, are more problematic. They can bring well-known psychological costs like anxiety and feeling down if one does badly. Preparing for public exams takes up a lot of time that could have been spent on immersion in worthwhile pursuits. As this preparation is often experienced as a form of hard, heteronomous work, it reinforces the work culture whose threat to well-being I have already dealt with. Sociologically, the public examination system tends to favour more affluent and education-savvy families. It thus also helps to reinforce the social divisions in well-being mentioned above.

If we start from the aim of a flourishing life for all, not just for some, there must be better ways of assessing learning. How can we find out how pupils are progressing in whole-hearted and successful involvement in worthwhile pursuits? Standard examinations tell us what they can do in exam conditions to display required knowledge in, say, mathematics. But good results may not tell us anything about their *attitudes* towards maths – about whether they love it or hate it. Standard examinations are not good at testing non-standard understanding like self-awareness or insight into human well-being. They are not good at testing aesthetic or interpersonal sensitivity, or indeed any of the dispositions discussed in 'The primacy of dispositions' on p. 131.

So how then *do* we assess progress in the well-being area? Those in the best position are not examiners for whom the pupil is simply a number, but people who know her well. Parents, for example. Parents do not have to *take steps* to find out how well their very young children are doing in speaking, being nice to their friends, getting stuck into things they enjoy. They pick this up from what they see and hear in everyday interactions with them. The evidence is *presented* to them: they do not have to seek it out. The same is true of the increasingly sophisticated connections that their children make in their understanding of the natural and social worlds.

In a well-conceived education system, the teacher's work is continuous with the parents'. This is especially true of the primary school, where children usually have the same teacher (plus teaching assistant) throughout the day. To some extent, primary teachers do not have to take steps to assess what children have learned. Like parents, they can pick this up from what they perceive around them. They see their pupils interacting co-operatively together on shared tasks. They gain a good idea from children's oral and written work of how their cognitive maps of the world are being built up. This informal monitoring is clearly not enough. Teachers deal with 30 children, not the parent's one or two. They need – and indeed use – some system of recording how every child is progressing, both for diagnostic reasons and because their pupils will soon be joining another teacher.

Secondary teachers are at a further remove from parents, at least in our current system. Even so, they can and do get a long way by everyday monitoring plus more systematic recording of progress and problems. The more orientated schools become to well-being, the more scope there will be for this.

Could records of achievement come to take the place of public exams in the upper secondary school? I see no reason why not. They are more in line with the world of whole-hearted engagement, and are able to celebrate this not only in academic fields but also in other types of endeavour. They do not lend themselves to competitive ranking, often on a national scale, nor the undesirable attitudes sometimes associated with this, like bitter striving for instrumental goods and feelings of superiority if successful, and of worthlessness if not. Provided there is some check on the competence and reliability of the teacher-recorder, records of achievement have a lot going for them.

One test of intrinsic commitment to a pursuit is whether the pursuer goes on with it when he or she does not have to. Public exams cannot test for this. For some secondary students, the work they do for their Spanish or chemistry exam is their last activity in the field. If they do well in it, what does this say about how much they love the subject? Imagine now someone who has studied elementary Spanish at school and a year or two after leaving it is getting deeper and deeper into Spanish literature and culture. That fact alone would be a good reason to think their time learning the subject at school was well spent.

The arguments in this section connect with what I wrote at the end of Chapter 15 on post-18 study at college or university. The influence of these institutions on the secondary school is huge. It is they that provide the rationale for most of the exam-orientated work we find in schools; and, via the demands of examining authorities, it is they that help to keep schools tightly within a culture of discrete subjects. The more the assumption is challenged that the ideal form of education is one that continues end-on to school into full-time higher education at 18 or 19, the easier will it become for schools to break free from the strangle-hold of current curriculum and assessment regimes.

Conclusion

More and more people are now asking what school education should be for. Britain and many other countries are saddled with a system that many do not want, but which, through inertia, is hard to remove. It is a system driven by demands beyond the school. These come not so much, as is often claimed, from 'the world of work' – employers are often loudest among those calling for schools to be more practically orientated and to give greater attention to personal qualities: they come more from university entrance requirements and parental aspirations for their children to meet them.

The hold that universities have on schools dates, in Britain, from the 1830s when the London Matriculation examination was introduced for admission to London University. In those days, that university still had a general course, based on encyclopaedic knowledge of academic disciplines. This explains why the new matriculation exam covered mathematics, natural philosophy (i.e. physics), chemistry, Greek and Latin, English language, outlines of history and geography, and (for honours) natural history.

Things are different now: universities run specialised degree courses. Yet they still insist on a close match between their own subjects of study and those examined at school. In addition, nearly two centuries of their matriculation and school certificate examinations have reinforced the notion that the school's main job is to teach a comprehensive range of academic disciplines.

Sometime in this twenty-first century we may break with this paradigm. We may come to agree that a curriculum devised for a horse-drawn age is no longer fit for purpose. If John Maynard Keynes is right in the main thrust of his prediction mentioned in the Introduction, our still newish century will see personal fulfilment trumping economic growth as a political objective, with the standard working week reduced in consequence. Schools, along with many other social institutions, will be transformed. Equipping everyone with the wherewithal for a flourishing personal and civic life will become their clear, unmuddied purpose.

I have written this book to help prepare for this transformation. Some may call the project utopian. It is not realistic, they may say, to expect school teachers, most of whom are specialists in some academic discipline, to step out into this unknown land of larger purposes. It is not realistic to expect university teachers to give up the power they now have to influence the secondary school curriculum, or to expect politicians to risk alienating parents, as well as those who work in schools and universities, by tampering with a system that provides a royal route for some to better-paid jobs and a comfortable life. Better than utopian dreaming, I will be told, is the pragmatic alternative of making sensible, small-scale changes where we can.

'Yeah, but . . . ,' as my little grandson has a habit of saying. If these small-scale changes are changes for the better, we must have some idea of what this 'better' involves. Without some notion of where we want to get to, how can we go forward at all? Possessing it is not incompatible with recognising obstacles in the path and with accepting that progress may be slow and irregular.

But who knows? Who would have imagined three or four decades ago that the struggle for women's rights would have made such headway, that the Soviet Empire and the apartheid regime in South Africa would both collapse?

The advent of the well-being school may be closer than we think.

Further reading

The account of well-being presented in this book owes a big debt to the writings of Joseph Raz. Chapter 12 of his *The Morality of Freedom* (1986) examines this concept, while Chapter 14 looks at its relationship with personal autonomy. Chapter 1 of *Ethics in the Public Domain* (1994) fills in more of the concept, while Chapters 6, 8 and 9 of *Engaging Reason* (1999) explore Raz's notion of the social dependence of values, and Chapter 13 is about the relationship between morality and self-interest. Finally, *The Practice of Value* (2003) develops the social dependence thesis further, with comments from Christine Korsgaard, Robert Pippin and Bernard Williams, plus a reply by Raz himself.

Part 1 of James Griffin's *Well-being* (1986) adjudicates between desire-satisfaction accounts and objective accounts of the concept, as well as looking at how morality relates to prudence. Both topics are also discussed in his *Value Judgement* (1996). Roger Crisp and Brad Hooker are editors of *Well-being and Morality: Essays in Honour of James Griffin* (2000). Its chapters attempt to clarify where Griffin stands on the desire theory versus objectivism issue and critically discuss his short list of central prudential values. The book also includes a reply by Griffin. Wayne Sumner's *Welfare, Happiness and Ethics* (1996) outlines central arguments for and against hedonism, objective theories and the desire theory. His own preferred alternative to these, the 'authentic happiness' view, sees well-being as a function of an autonomous individual's satisfaction with his or her life.

Human Flourishing (1999) is a collection edited by E.F. Paul, F.D. Miller and J. Paul. It includes, among other contributions, an essay by Charles Larmore arguing against the idea of a life plan as a necessary feature of flourishing, and Richard Arneson's critique of desire satisfaction accounts. *The Market: Ethics, Knowledge and Politics* (1998), by John O'Neill, links market theory with desire satisfaction accounts and argues against these in favour of an objectivist account based on an Aristotelian approach to human nature.

Two recent defences of a hedonistic view of well-being are Fred Feldman's *Pleasure and the Good Life* (2004) and Roger Crisp's *Reasons and the Good*

(2006). For further discussion of secular views on the meaning of life and moral values, see Richard Norman's *On Humanism* (2004).

Picking up from the discussion of dispositions in Part 2 Chapter 16, there is a good account of the virtues of reflectiveness, perspective and self-knowledge in Tiberius (2003: chs 3–5).

On education for flourishing in the context of a more comprehensive account of educational aims, see Harry Brighouse's *On Education* (2006). Also relevant is the educational chapter (8) of Robin Barrow's *Happiness* (1980). I discuss problems with life planning in White (1990: 85–9). There are fuller discussions of well-being aims of education to do with religion, work, morality, the market, and patriotism in Part 3 of White (2005).

References

Barrow, R. (1980) *Happiness*. Oxford: Martin Robertson.

Beadle, P. (2010) *How to Teach*. Carmarthen: Crown House.

Bennett, J. (1830) *History of Tewkesbury*. London: Longman.

Brighouse, H. (2006) *On Education*. London: Routledge.

Burleigh, M. (2000) *The Third Reich*. London: Macmillan.

Chitty, C. (2007) *Eugenics, Race and Intelligence in Education*. London: Continuum.

Clarke, F. (1923) *Essays in the Politics of Education*. Oxford: Oxford University Press.

Comenius, J. A. (1638/1907) *The Great Didactic* (trans. Keatinge, M. W.). London: Adam and Charles Black.

Conway, D. (2010) *Liberal Education and the National Curriculum*. London: Civitas.

Crisp, R (2006) *Reasons and the Good*. Oxford: Oxford University Press.

Crisp, R. and Hooker, B. (eds) (2000) *Well-being and Morality: Essays in Honour of James Griffin*. Oxford: Oxford University Press.

DCSF (2008) *The Role of the School in Promoting Pupil Well-being*. London: HMSO.

DfEE/QCA (1999) *The National Curriculum Handbook for Teachers in England*. London: HMSO.

Feldman, F. (2004) *Pleasure and the Good Life*. Oxford: Oxford University Press.

Galton, F. (1978) *Hereditary Genius* (reprint of 1892 edition, first published 1869). London: Friedmann.

Griffin, J. (1986) *Well-being*. Oxford: Oxford University Press.

Griffin, J. (1996) *Value Judgement*. Oxford: Oxford University Press.

Hirsch, F. (1977) *Social Limits to Growth*. London: Routledge and Kegan Paul.

Husbands, C., Kitson, A. and Pendry, A. (2003) *Understanding History Teaching*. Maidenhead: Open University Press.

Layard, R. (2005) *Happiness: Lessons from a New Science*. London: Penguin.

Macintyre, A. (1981) *After Virtue*. London: Duckworth.

Mill, J. S. (1861) *Utilitarianism* (1993 edition). London: Everyman.

Moore, G. E. (1903) *Principia Ethica*. Cambridge: Cambridge University Press.

Morgan, E. S. (1944) *The Puritan Family*. Boston, MA: Trustees of the Public Library.

Mosley, C. (ed.) (2007) *The Mitfords: Letters Between Six Sisters*. London: Fourth Estate.

Norman, R. (2004) *On Humanism*. London: Routledge.

O'Neill, J. (1998) *The Market: Ethics, Knowledge and Politics*. London: Routledge.

Parfit, D. (1984) *Reasons and Persons*. Oxford: Clarendon Press.

Paul, E. F., Miller F. D. and Paul, J. (eds) (1999) *Human Flourishing*. Cambridge: Cambridge University Press.

Peters, R. S. (1966) *Ethics and Education*. London: Allen and Unwin.

Rawls, J (1971) *A Theory of Justice*. Oxford: Oxford University Press.

Raz, J. (1986) *The Morality of Freedom*. Oxford: Oxford University Press.

Raz, J. (1994) *Ethics in the Public Domain*. Oxford: Oxford University Press.

Raz, J. (1999) *Engaging Reason*. Oxford: Oxford University Press.

Raz, J. (2003) *The Practice of Value*. Oxford: Oxford University Press.

Seligman *et al.* (2009) 'Positive education'. *Oxford Review of Education*.

Skidelsky, R. (2009) 'How much money is enough?' *The Guardian*, 23 November.

Suissa, J. (2008) 'Lessons from a new science? On teaching happiness in schools'. *Journal of Philosophy of Education*, 42, 3/4.

Sumner, W. (1996) *Welfare, Happiness and Ethics*. Oxford: Oxford University Press.

Tawney, R. H. (1926) *Religion and the Rise of Capitalism*. West Drayton: Penguin.

Tiberius, V. (2008) *The Reflective Life: Living Wisely within Our Limits*. Oxford: Oxford University Press.

Weber, M. (1930) *The Protestant Ethic and the Spirit of Capitalism*. London: Allen and Unwin.

Wesley, J. (1749) 'A short account of the school in Kingswood', in Ives, A. G. (1970) *Kingswood School in Wesley's Day and Since*. London: Epworth, pp. 11–18.

White, J. (1990) *Education and the Good Life*. London: Kogan Page.

White, J. (2005) *The Curriculum and the Child: The Selected Works of John White*. London: Routledge.

White, J. (2009) 'Further and higher: a philosophical divide?', in Garrod, N. and Macfarlane, B. (eds) *Challenging Boundaries: Managing the Integration of Post-secondary Education*. London: Routledge.

White, J. (forthcoming) *The Invention of the Secondary Curriculum*. London: Palgrave Macmillan.

Wilkinson, R. and Pickett, K. (2010) *The Spirit Level: Why Equality is Better for Everyone*. London: Penguin.

Williams, B. (1976) 'Persons, character and morality', in Rorty, A. (ed.) *The Identity of Persons*. Berkeley, CA: University of California Press.

Williams, B. (1985) *Ethics and the Limits of Philosophy*. London: Fontana.

Index

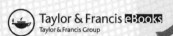